Working with Infertility and Grief

Working with Infertility and Grief: A Practical Guide for Helping Professionals explores issues of grief, including disenfranchised grief and chronic sorrow, related to infertility and reproductive loss. Out of the small handful of books related to this topic, this is the first of its kind geared toward equipping helping professionals who assist those grieving unrecognized losses. Written through the lens of the literary framework of The Hero's Journey, this comprehensive practitioner guide directly targets mental health professionals working with clients, supervisees, or students who have experienced infertility, miscarriage, or death of an infant. This book is also for those who experienced it themselves. Readers will learn more about the crisis of infertility and reproductive loss, gain insight into the experience of those suffering, and acquire practical tools and strategies for helping and healing. This text is broad enough to be integrated into a course for a graduate program and specific enough to serve as a shelf reference for those in practice.

Whitney L. Jarnagin, PhD, is the dean of behavioral and social sciences and professor of psychology at Walters State Community College in Morristown, Tennessee.

Denis' A. Thomas, PhD, is an author, podcaster, adjunct professor, conference presenter, homeschool teacher, and freelance writer.

Megan C. Herscher, PhD, is the coordinator and associate professor of clinical mental health counseling at Carson-Newman University. She provides post-graduate supervision through her firm Herscher Consultation.

Working with Infertility and Grief

A Practical Guide for Helping Professionals

Whitney L. Jarnagin,
Denis' A. Thomas, and
Megan C. Herscher

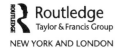
Routledge
Taylor & Francis Group

NEW YORK AND LONDON

Designed cover image: © Getty Images

First published 2024
by Routledge
605 Third Avenue, New York, NY 10158

and by Routledge
4 Park Square, Milton Park, Abingdon, Oxon, OX14 4RN

Routledge is an imprint of the Taylor & Francis Group, an informa business

ISBN: 978-1-032-36796-5 (hbk)
ISBN: 978-1-032-36792-7 (pbk)
ISBN: 978-1-003-33640-2 (ebk)

DOI: 10.4324/9781003336402

Typeset in Helvetica
by MPS Limited, Dehradun

Contents

About the Authors

Dr. Whitney Jarnagin is the dean of behavioral and social sciences and professor of psychology at Walters State Community College in Morristown, TN. A graduate of the counselor education program at the University of Tennessee, she is a National Certified Counselor (NCC) and licensed school counselor for grades PreK-12 in the state of Tennessee. Her research interests include wellness and women's issues. Noted accomplishments include receiving the Distinguished Faculty Member Award at Walters State, securing four Tennessee Board of Regents course revitalization grants, several publications, and numerous presentations on topics related to counseling, teaching, and learning. She enjoys spending time with her family, reading, and doing just about anything outdoors. A counselor at heart, she loves educating the next generation of helping professionals. She and her family live in Russellville, TN.

Dr. Denis' (pronounced Denise) Thomas is a former mental health counseling associate professor. She created a play therapy specialization and served as the first faculty director of the Center for Play Therapy and Expressive Arts at Lipscomb University. She hosted two podcasts: *Play Therapy Across the Lifespan* and *Wellness with Dr. Denis'*. She has authored or co-authored seven books, including *Creative Play Therapy with Adolescents and Adults: Moving from Helping to Healing*, *Wellness That Works: How to Create a Wellness Plan*, and *Overcoming Challenges: Making Your Wellness Plan Work* along with a cookbook, book chapters, and more than 20 academic journal and magazine articles. She has presented at international, national, and other conferences more than 30 times. Dr. Denis' was an Outstanding Teacher nominee in 2018. She earned a Ph.D. from the University of Tennessee and was a National Certified Counselor

(NCC) and a licensed professional counselor (LPC). She lives with her husband and homeschools their three children in Nashville, TN.

Dr. Megan Herscher serves as associate professor of clinical mental health counseling and coordinator of the clinical mental health program at Carson-Newman University and is the sole proprietor of her supervision and consultation firm Herscher Consultation, LLC. She recently transitioned from the position of president of the Tennessee Licensed Professional Counselor's Association to past president in June of 2022. Other professional roles have included president of Chi Sigma Iota at the University of Tennessee, president of the Smoky Mountain Counseling Association, and president of the Tennessee Clinical Mental Health Association as well as a leadership role in the Tennessee Association for Counselor Education and Supervision (TACES). Dr. Herscher holds the license of LPC-MHSP (licensed professional counseling with a mental health services provider designation) in the state of Tennessee and LPC (licensed professional counselor) in Washington, DC, and is a designated supervisor with the state of Tennessee. Additionally, she is credentialed by the NBCC as a National Certified Counselor (NCC) and approved clinical supervisor (ACC). She resides in Knoxville, TN, with her husband and three success stories (children).

Acknowledgments

To the Sovereign Lord whose thoughts and ways are higher than mine … thank you that my pain had a purpose. To Bradley, my number one cheerleader and fan, you were the only one who stood by me during the storm. And to our one-shot wonder, we are so very grateful for you.

I am grateful to my co-authors who continue to teach me that my weaknesses are my strengths, and my strengths are my weaknesses, making me better for both. Thank you to my husband Tim who was a steadfast anchor in the storm of infertility and for the three gifts that came from it. I am also grateful for the Lipscomb writer's group – Dr. Holly Allen, Dr. Donita Brown, Dr. Tessa Sanders, and Dr. Leanne Smith – who encouraged both the writing and the writer.

I'd like to acknowledge my husband and best friend Adam, my family for putting up with me throughout the writing process, and of course the "aunties".

Many thanks to our Carson-Newman graduate assistants, Meredith Ginn and Rebecca Gomez, for the many hours of work you put in.

Thanks to Dr. Melanie Morris who teaches her students and colleagues the most thorough case conceptualization which we used as a template.

Many thanks to Dr. Ginger W. Carter, MD, FACOG, for reviewing and providing feedback on the biological aspects of infertility in Chapter 2. You are a gifted physician and a special friend.

Thank you to Joseph Campbell for first identifying the Hero's Journey and influencing generations of writers, even nonfiction writers.

Thanks to all the brave heroes who contributed their stories to the vignettes used throughout the book. Your experiences with infertility and reproductive loss made the content come to life for our readers.

We also want to acknowledge those we asked to share stories but who declined because the pain was still too present. We are rooting for you as you continue to heal. Your journey isn't over yet.

Figures

Introduction

What Is the Hero's Journey?

Why would we want to write a book about infertility, and what do religious and mythological stories have to do with it?

All three of us have traveled the journey of infertility. We have experienced decades of waiting for the children we longed to hold. We know the Mother's Day melancholy, the changes in our marriages, and the minefield of family comments. We have lived with an inability to conceive and secondary infertility. We have paid for the medications, hormones, and procedures. We've had discussions with our doctors about possible options and tried many of them.

We have personally experienced the griefs that accompany this journey. We know the pain of miscarriages, failed in vitro attempts, and medical procedures that did not work. We have grieved our bodies not working, despaired with spiraling thoughts, and felt social isolation as others' growing families left us behind. Although we are in the last phase of our personal journeys, they are not fully over yet.

We are also all three counselor educators. We are the professors who teach the counseling and psychological research that helps people heal from these kinds of wounds. We are living in a place where knowledge and personal experience intersect. So, we should have all the answers, right? We really wish that were true. We don't have all the answers, but we do have some, and we want to share what we have learned with you.

In fact, education and the journey of infertility is how we know each other and what made this writing project possible. Whitney and Denis' (pronounced Denise) met at the University of Tennessee while pursuing doctoral degrees and while Denis' was undergoing infertility treatments. As friends, they talked about the hope Denis' had of finding a new doctor and the joy of getting

DOI: 10.4324/9781003336402-1

pregnant, but they grieved over a miscarriage between teaching classes and drafting dissertations.

A few years later, Whitney and Megan (who was also a UT graduate) were asked to teach counseling courses as adjunct faculty at their alma mater. The coordinator of the program hosted a gathering for full-time and adjunct faculty so they could connect with one another and discuss class-related issues prior to the beginning of the semester. Children were invited, and Whitney noticed that Megan had an only child just like she did. Little did they know at the time, both women were struggling with secondary infertility.

Months later, Whitney, still in the middle of her journey, was desperate for someone to talk to. She cornered Megan at a local conference and asked questions about her own path to parenthood. Megan confirmed that she had also struggled with infertility. It was a relief for Whitney, knowing she wasn't alone. And it was refreshing discussing the heartache and pain of infertility with someone who had been there, too.

Then, one fateful summer day, Whitney and Denis' met at a pool near Nashville so their elementary-aged kids could swim together while they caught up. Denis' was aware of Whitney's infertility, but they had never discussed it in-depth because they had been out of touch the years following graduation. Denis', as most good friends (and helping professionals) do, put on her counselor hat and talked with Whitney about her struggle. As part of that conversation, she asked the most poignant question: "What do you need now?" That was a turning point for Whitney. She realized she had been so focused on trying to build a family and so grief-stricken with the process and result that she had completely neglected to consider what might come next. The answer? A new purpose. And part of that purpose included using her pain to help others.

Whitney had the idea of writing journal articles to educate helping professionals about how to work with clients facing infertility. She and Denis' thought a third perspective would be beneficial. Whitney remembered Megan and asked if she'd like to help. Megan was all in, and after a few meetings wrestling with what they wanted to write about and where they might submit their work, Megan said, "I'm tired of writing articles. Let's write a book!"

So, we wrote a book. This book. It's one way to make sense of our personal suffering, but it's also what we do. We teach. We share knowledge. We encourage. We train counselors. We help people heal from deep wounds. We wanted to use our skills in empathy, educating, and easing pain to aid professional helpers as they work with clients experiencing infertility.

What does any of that have to do with a Hero's Journey? In literature and movies, the story structure of the Hero's Journey is often used to explain how the protagonist is thrust into the journey, forever changed, and then returned to the old life, a different person. It's a great analogy for the story of infertility, too. Isn't that what happened to us? We were thrust into a journey we didn't want to take, it left us forever changed, and then we had to figure out what to do with it all. During that journey, we taught students who also struggled with infertility, and we supervised counselors who were helping clients with infertility. Some of our supervisees struggled with infertility, too. Forever looking for ways to teach concepts in memorable ways so students retain the knowledge, we wondered how we could take our personal experiences and combine them with our professional experiences. The book you are holding is the answer to that. It's our combined experience, research, and wisdom, mixed with a story structure, and we hope it gives you some answers, too.

When working with a person experiencing infertility, no one knows how the story will end. Most of this book is written for professional helpers. That's the term we'll use throughout the book for the counselor, psychologist, social worker, marriage and family therapist, and anyone else who provides mental health services to clients. But if you, the professional helper, are also on the journey of infertility, it will help you as well.

We like simple, memorable steps, so we share three phases of the journey. We can all remember three things at a time, right? Within each phase are four to six stages if you'd like a deeper dive into the smaller steps. This will give you a practical way to honor client stories by viewing infertility as a journey and your clients as unlikely – and possibly unwilling – heroes.

It is helpful to understand common patterns and themes that your client will likely experience along the way, which allows you to have a better understanding of what has already happened, clarify the distress in the present, and prepare her for the future. While the pattern of every journey has similarities for all clients, we must emphasize that each story is different, and multiple ending options exist. The most practical suggestion we have is to honor your client's individual story from her perspective.

THE HERO'S JOURNEY

Joseph Campbell outlined what is perhaps the most iconic story structure from literature in the book *The Hero with 1,000 Faces* (2004), originally published in 1949. Drawing from his studies in mythology and religion, Campbell noticed that the protagonist followed a predictable story structure (at least in well-written stories) which allowed for many variations with similar story patterns. Even 75 years after the publication of his book, this story structure shapes most epic movies, novels, and stories today.

In a later interview series that aired on PBS in 1988 (Campbell & Moyers, 1991), Campbell explained that the Hero's Journey is a universal experience. This means it applies to the stories of our lives, not just fiction writing, and it can, therefore, be applied to client stories of infertility. Having a framework for understanding the tremendous amount of information received from clients helps us to clarify the experience and anticipate what is to come.

Our goal is to adapt Campbell's story structure into something that is easily memorable during a client session with a hero struggling with infertility. We've changed the language and condensed some of the stages to better fit client therapy, but the original ideas are from Campbell's work. Some clients and therapists may enjoy the language and particulars of the Hero's Journey and apply all the stages in detail, but others may use it more loosely to understand the journey from a big-picture, three-phase perspective. Just as each journey is unique, the work you do with each client will be unique. While acknowledging that all genders embark on this journey, we recognize that most of the clients, supervisees, and students that this book is geared towards helping will identify as female. For simplicity and ease of reading, we will use feminine pronouns but continue to use Campbell's language of the Hero's Journey and refer to the female protagonist as the hero.

In every hero's journey, the main character is introduced and somehow presented with the journey in the Separation Phase of the story. For the story of infertility, this is the point that the client is faced with an inability to have something she deeply desires: children, or more children if experiencing secondary infertility. This stage separates what used to be from what is yet to be.

Next, in the Quest Phase, the hero faces challenges that forever change her. For clients struggling with infertility, this might include any combination of natural, medical, or court options in an attempt to build a family. She faces limitations of her body, spiritual questions, mental challenges, and emotional obstacles on the road of trials. She is tempted to end the quest. Yet, she encounters guides and other characters who help her continue.

Finally, in the Return Phase, the hero reenters her previous world in this changed state, and she discovers that she does not fit in as she did before. Maybe she accepts living without natural children. She may interact with those who never experienced infertility. Perhaps the family she started this journey to attain does not live up to the idealized, fairytale-like ending. See Figure 0.1 for the three phases of the Hero's Journey. Next, let's break these phases into smaller stages to understand the Hero's Journey in more detail.

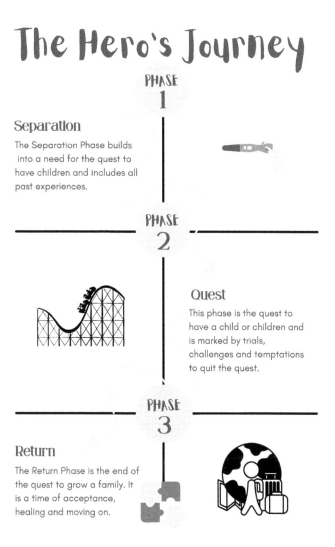

The Hero's Journey

PHASE 1

Separation

The Separation Phase builds into a need for the quest to have children and includes all past experiences.

PHASE 2

Quest

This phase is the quest to have a child or children and is marked by trials, challenges and temptations to quit the quest.

PHASE 3

Return

The Return Phase is the end of the quest to grow a family. It is a time of acceptance, healing and moving on.

FIGURE 0.1 The Hero's Journey of Infertility

THE SEPARATION PHASE

The Separation Phase, where the journey begins, makes the journey necessary. The beginning of the story likely happens in childhood as identities about children, motherhood, and career form. It may include previous trauma narratives that are not directly related to infertility but impact the client's understanding of her world. However, at some point, there becomes a need to embark on the Hero's Journey of infertility.

In therapeutic terms, the basic story begins with a person or couple that desires to start a family but cannot. At this point, a decision is made to stay in the same place or embark on the journey to find a solution and have children, but this is a false choice. If the hero opts to, say, pursue medical treatment, she is proactively choosing to start the journey. But, if she decides to passively wait for change to happen, she is still a traveler on the journey. The distinction of having or lacking autonomy about what happens is important, and it teaches you something about your hero's character.

The Separation Phase begins even before your client embarks on the quest of infertility, and it contains all her natural strengths, experiences, and vulnerabilities that she brings with her on the journey. It includes how she starts trying to have children, resistance to some options, and rising discontent. Your client recognizes the need for help to have children, but she may or may not be seeking your services at this time. If you want more detail, the Separation Phase has five stages (See Figure 0.2).

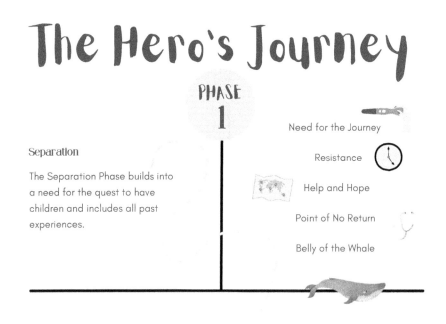

FIGURE 0.2 The Separation Phase of the Hero's Journey of Infertility

Need for the Journey

This stage is all that precedes your client's call to action. Campbell describes it as the motivation for the journey that makes it impossible for the hero to refuse. With infertility, what she has been doing to start or increase her family has not worked, so she recognizes that some sort of a journey may be needed, although she likely hopes it will not. This is when your client will likely start seeking information or first learns that outside intervention is necessary. However, this stage builds from light information gathering and hoping things will work out to a clear understanding that the quest for children is necessary.

For many clients, the very act of trying to release the hope to have a family increases it instead, and this strong desire for children makes the call impossible to refuse. Though she may strongly wish to avoid the journey – the medical appointments, the cost, the medication, the procedures, the legal fees, and the unknown – her family as she dreams it is threatened, so she becomes compelled to accept the challenge and the interruptions to life as she knows it.

Resistance

Campbell recognized in his studies of heroic stories that the listener, reader, or viewer needed to understand the conflict around embarking on the journey. The journey will become very difficult later, so you must understand why it is so important when the trials come. You will probably see this with a client who has recognized the need for the journey, but she second-guesses it and takes a step back. She does not want to embark on the journey and declines in some way, maybe even overtly refusing. Her fears set in about what this journey means. The adoptive mother might not select her. The in vitro process might not work. The hormone injections might negatively impact her career. Her husband might find someone else who can carry his child. She may feel defective or weak. She may try every option possible and still not bring a baby home to the nursery. These fears create her resistance to the journey. Without a strong enough motivation for the quest, your client may take a break from trying. The options and stress probably feel over-whelming.

Help and Hope

In Campbell's description (2004), help comes from a supernatural source, such as an angel, wizard, or deity, that enters the story briefly, but your hero may find help from more common sources. She finds a guide or a mentor who helps her identify a tool she needs to embark on this infertility journey. Fellow characters on the journey are part of each phase, but they provide different things in each phase as the hero transforms. In the Separation Phase, one important tool fellow characters provide is hope. Other tools include information, inspiration from other people's journeys, and possibly learning about options of which she was previously unaware. These tools could be from a book, a support group, or a new friend who also experienced infertility. Guides may also be professional experts in infertility. While this aid could come from a variety of sources, it is likely to be a source that has entered her life recently and does not remain constant. You are certainly one of her guides on this journey if you are working with her during the Separation Phase.

Point of No Return

This is the point when the quest to overcome infertility officially begins. This is when "infertility" becomes the diagnosis, the appointment is made with a medical specialist or lawyer, or the search for a surrogate begins in earnest. It is the point when things change, and she steps away from what she knows to move into uncertainty and ambiguity. It is often a teetering blend of joyful hope and fearful ambiguity. She questions if it is the right or best thing, and she may still harbor the secret hope that she will get pregnant naturally. But staying in the same place is no longer an option. This is when, usually unknown to the client, that change from *before* infertility to *after* infertility happens, and things will never return to the way they were.

Belly of the Whale

Campbell (2004) called this stage of the Hero's Journey the belly of the whale, and it is a reference to the Biblical story of the Israelite judge Jonah who refused a call to preach to the people of the enemy city of Nineveh. He instead bought a fare on a boat going the opposite direction, and after a terrible storm where he instructed the crew to throw him overboard, he was swallowed by a big fish and then regurgitated on land to continue his journey to Nineveh. For our hero, like Jonah, the belly marks the point when the journey is unavoidable, despite her unwillingness or fears to embark on it. It may seem that forces greater than her are at work, and this first difficult obstacle of the journey is when she begins to change noticeably. She is now aware that she is separating from who she was pre-infertility, and she accepts that the journey is inevitable.

THE QUEST PHASE

The second phase, the Quest, is marked by challenges. This is probably the phase when she will seek your skills to help her. One part of this phase is aptly called the Road of Trials, and these challenges continue to transform the hero, often in unanticipated ways. While the word *transformation* sounds hopeful, this stage is often characterized by bouts of hopelessness.

She experiences heartache, disappointment, and anger and may be tempted to give up the mission. She questions if it is worth it. While parts of this journey are traveled in solitude, an important aspect of the Quest Phase is the support from the people she meets along the way. These include medical professionals, friends who have also experienced infertility, and various guides (which include you, the professional helper). During the Quest, she may meet birth mothers, social workers, and legal professionals. She may encounter experts who have written books, conducted research, or authored blog posts. The one certainty with infertility is that it feels like a roller coaster with thrilling highs and stomach-churning lows. Hope soars and disappointment devastates, and in between, she waits. See Figure 0.3 for the stages in the Quest phase.

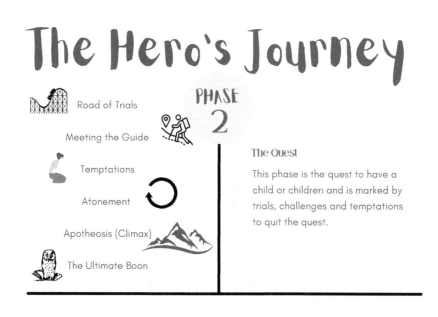

FIGURE 0.3 The Quest Phase of the Hero's Journey of Infertility

The Road of Trials

This phase is just what it sounds like, a series of challenges. In the story, our hero learns skills, is strengthened, and grows in confidence, but the challenges lead to the transformation, and the hero will fail some or most of these. With infertility, failed trials are markers of the hero not being pregnant, things such as starting her period, a negative pregnancy test, or a miscarriage. Each effort or procedure that is not successful is part of the road of trials. The road is grueling and hard, often watered with many tears. This part of the journey is often what brings her to you.

Meeting the Guide

The original title for this stage, The Meeting with the Goddess, came from Campbell's work with mythology literature, which included supernatural elements. For the client experiencing infertility, it is unlikely she will find herself walking through a forest and meeting a beautiful creature bathed in bright light who helps her continue her journey. However, she may have a chance encounter with someone outside of her periphery who points the way to a previously unavailable solution, such as embryo donation, international adoption, or funding that may change the course of her journey. If you are beginning your work with the client during the Quest Phase, you may be this encouraging guide, especially if you have expertise working with infertility.

Temptations

This stage is patterned by the siren call of Greek mythology, luring sailors to their death and longed-for relief. Relief is the keyword. Your client has been hurting for a while now, and she may be engulfed in negative emotions. She strongly desires relief from the pain. Clients will likely hit a point where they are tempted to abandon their quest, not because they do not want to succeed in the quest of having a baby, but because they need a respite from hurting. Some will quit temporarily and others permanently. Your client may dissolve her relationship with her partner or fantasize about what it would be like to do so. She might use substances, food, or self-harm to cope. The temptation could be anything that might end the pain of the journey, even if the consequences are high.

Atonement

Campbell called this stage Atonement, and it highlights the transformational aspect of this stage. This pivotal plot point is when your client recognizes the true purpose of her journey was not simply the quest to have a baby. This is the culmination of the transformation when she faces the conflict with the person or entity that holds power in her life. She has already experienced many battles around her lack of control, her body, her circumstances, and her outcomes. This stage is often spiritual and existential, but unlike previous wrestling with those kinds of questions, your client finds answers here, including a higher purpose in her suffering. Rarely in real life is this stage as dramatic as in movies, but clients that heal from infertility must come to grips with their personal lack of control over the situation and with whom or where they believe that control lies. This is also when the client realizes that the journey was not really about having a baby – the perceived goal for the journey up until now – but about what she has gained and become because of the journey and the other lives that are impacted by it.

Apotheosis

According to the Encyclopedia Britannica, (Britannica, 2019) Apotheosis is a Greek word that means to deify, but you probably know it as the climax of the story. Building on the wisdom and purpose achieved in the Atonement Stage, the client uses this for ultimate success on the journey. Regardless of the actual family result, the client makes peace with (and achieves ultimate victory over) infertility. None of the possible outcomes of growing a family are the end of the story. Instead, this stage is the meaning behind why the journey was even necessary for your client. Without that personal and individual answer, she will not ultimately succeed in healing from the journey, so she may still have a battle to find it. In psychological terms, this is the cognitive work of assigning meaning and understanding.

The Ultimate Boon

In ancient mythology, this phase often included the acquiring of a magical item, but for your client, it is the acquiring of wisdom and understanding, which could feel magical. The boon is coming to terms with infertility on an emotional level. It is the final step of the Quest Phase, the relief after the transformation in the Atonement Stage, and the full realization of what transformation means in the Apotheosis Stage. Finally, your client experiences peace after the battle … but this temporary respite is not the end of her journey.

THE RETURN PHASE

Entering the Return Phase marks the end of the quest, but not the end of the journey. Regardless of the outcome of the quest, the hero must now reassemble her life. The consuming focus is no longer on having a baby, and she is not the same person as she was when she started this journey. She has experienced a tumult of emotions, and many of those may not yet be resolved. She has made career and life decisions during her journey that have lingering positive and negative consequences, and she needs to come to peace with those choices. This is the meaning-making that you help your clients realize.

Her relationships have changed, especially with her partner if she has one. She and her partner may move into the relationship challenges that come with young children without ever addressing how their sexual relationship changed while trying to conceive. One or both of them may carry guilt for being on the journey. Family and social relationships changed as well. Peers may be years into having children and be in a different phase of life now. In-laws may have invested money in treatment or adoption fees, and they may have unwelcome opinions about your client's choices at the end of the quest.

The hero may still be grieving a miscarriage, stillbirth, or the lost years of infertility. She may live with more fear because she has experienced reproductive losses. She may have a friend or family member who had a similar due date to her lost child, and now she navigates watching that child grow up, each birthday a marker of a year her own child did not get. The baby may have an unwelcome diagnosis that shadows and challenges what was expected to be a joyous addition to the family. She may also have regrets or wish she had done things differently.

Now as she returns, she could be hesitant. She may physically move closer to family, or it may be a more symbolic return, a getting back to normal. Your client could seek or experience a change that makes it impossible to return to "before" – a divorce, a move, or a career change – yet she still must reintegrate.

Return may be reintegrating or reinventing herself, but the key difference is that the quest to have a baby has ended. As she returns, whatever that return looks like in her story, she will continue to have challenges. Although this phase may be marked by a period of rest from the quest, what could be unrecognized is that this is the time for healing from the journey. Unfortunately, many clients quit the journey before they do this. Moving on is not healing, which is why your role in her story is so important. See Figure 0.4 for the stages in the Return Phase.

Refusal of the Return

In this stage, your client recognizes that she cannot return to the ways things were before infertility because she is not that woman anymore. She recognizes

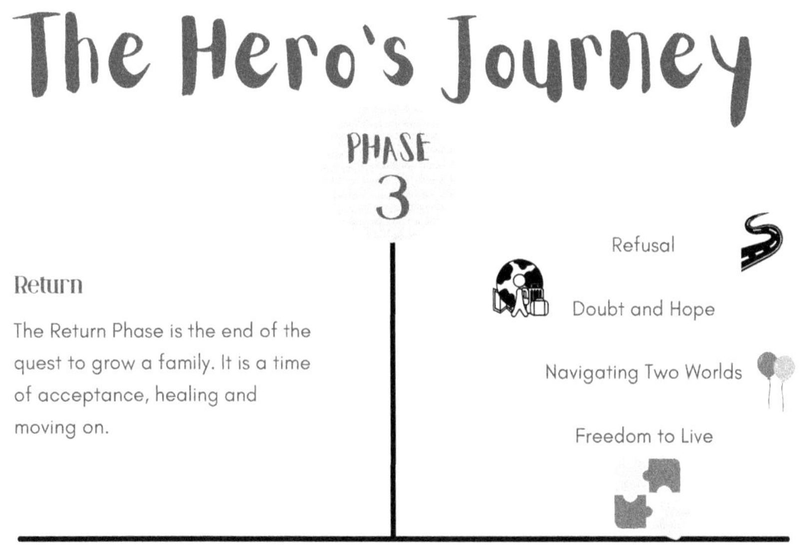

The Hero's Journey

PHASE
3

Return

The Return Phase is the end of the quest to grow a family. It is a time of acceptance, healing and moving on.

Refusal

Doubt and Hope

Navigating Two Worlds

Freedom to Live

FIGURE 0.4 The Return Phase of the Hero's Journey of Infertility

that those who have not experienced infertility will not understand her journey and may be insensitive to it. She may also notice that she easily identifies others who are struggling to have children even before she hears their stories. It includes a sense of not fitting back into her former life. For some, the return might be a literal move back home closer to family support. For some, it may be recognizing that her growth and change on this journey are different than her partner's. In this stage, she recognizes that her life post-quest is not as easy as she thought it would be.

Doubt and Hope

While we love happy, neat endings, the reality is that the ghosts of infertility may still haunt your client. Even with an acceptance of the journey and recognition of the strengths she has gained from the journey, your client will still have times of resentfulness and bitterness that she had to experience the journey at all. She will wrestle with the powers that have control again and question whether it really was worth it given the emotional scars she now carries. For clients with postpartum depression, children with medical concerns, or a partner that leaves the relationship, they may revisit previous doubts and insecurities. Clients may desire to avoid, numb, or escape again.

Although infertility is an isolating journey, it is not a solitary one. It doesn't need to be. Just as your client found help from a guide during the Separation and Quest Phases, she finds help from a guide again to get her home. This is a third opportunity for you to be the guide, but she will also find other guides, those who help her get home metaphorically. You'll notice a resurfacing of hope and an increased motivation to continue this journey.

Navigating Two Worlds

In this phase, she integrates. Here the client officially returns to a new normal. She has her hard-won wisdom, she has battled the fears that still haunt her, and she has identified sources of help. Now she returns, despite how changed she is. It may be with celebration or with sadness. She knows she has overcome, and she can see the pre-journey life through a different lens. She returns with wisdom, strength, and understanding. She also bears sorrow, pain, and loss that she did not possess before. She has sacrificed her idealism, optimism, and blind trust for wisdom, realism, and faith. She has completed her journey with unanticipated positive and negative consequences, yet she has peace.

Freedom to Live

After the difficult journey, the road of trials, the realization that this journey was not only about the quest to have a baby, and the return, the hero has finally earned the freedom to live in comfort and peace. She experiences this internally and externally. She may have other journeys to embark upon (after all, good stories have sequels), but this journey (if processed to completion) ends with freedom. It is a satisfying, if not the idealized, perfect ending. Your role as the professional helper was likely essential in getting her all the way to this last stage.

CONCLUSION

That is the Hero's Journey applied to infertility. As you can see, each client you work with will have a unique story, but her journey will still follow this general story structure. Her plot twists and battles are personal to her, but they follow this broad pattern so that you can anticipate some of the setbacks. We believe that the three broad phases – Separation, Quest, and Return – are sufficient to help most clients, and there is value in using frameworks that fit easily in working memory (three phases are easily remembered). However, becoming familiar with the 15 stages within those phases will enhance your ability to assist your clients struggling with infertility all the way to the end of their journeys. See Figure 0.5 for a list of the three phases along with the 15 stages.

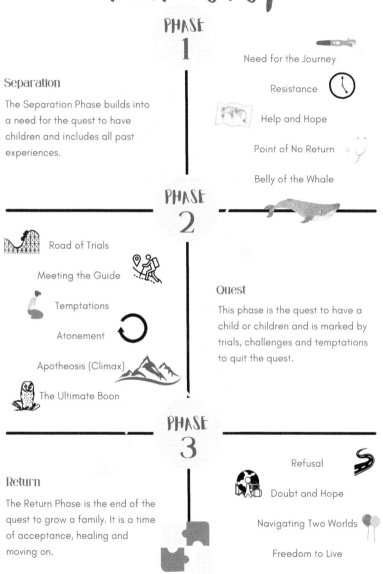

The Hero's Journey
of Infertility

PHASE 1

Separation

The Separation Phase builds into a need for the quest to have children and includes all past experiences.

Need for the Journey

Resistance

Help and Hope

Point of No Return

Belly of the Whale

PHASE 2

Road of Trials

Meeting the Guide

Temptations

Atonement

Apotheosis (Climax)

The Ultimate Boon

Quest

This phase is the quest to have a child or children and is marked by trials, challenges and temptations to quit the quest.

PHASE 3

Return

The Return Phase is the end of the quest to grow a family. It is a time of acceptance, healing and moving on.

Refusal

Doubt and Hope

Navigating Two Worlds

Freedom to Live

FIGURE 0.5 The Hero's Journey of Infertility with 15 Phases

In Neil Gaiman's (2002) novella *Coraline*, he paraphrased a quotation from author G.K. Chesterton stating that fairy tales let us know dragons exist but that they can also be beaten. As we apply the ideas of Joseph Campbell to working with clients struggling with the dragon of infertility, we want to encourage you that dragons can be beaten, and a seemingly hopeless, never-ending journey can have a good ending.

Whitney Jarnagin

Denis' Thomas

Megan Herscher

REFERENCES

Britannica, T. Editors of Encyclopedia (2019, November 7). *Apotheosis*. Encyclopedia Britannica. Retrieved October 4, 2022, from https://www.britannica.com/topic/apotheosis

Campbell J. (1949). *The hero with a thousand faces*. Pantheon.

Campbell, J. (2004). *The hero with a thousand faces*. Princeton, NJ: Princeton University Press.

Campbell, J., & Moyers, B. (1991). *Power of myth*. Bantam Doubleday Dell Publishing Group.

Gaiman, N. (2002). *Coraline*. Bloomsbury Publishing PLC.

PART ONE

The Biopsychosocial Crisis of Infertility

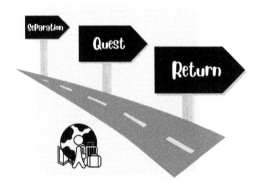

DOI: 10.4324/9781003336402-2

.

CHAPTER ONE

The Diagnosis

So, You Can't Have a Baby: What's the Big Deal?

Infertility.

For so many people, it's just a word. But for those affected, it carries a punch that hits hard and low and leaves lasting effects. Why did we write this book? We want you to know how deep and long and wide and complex the experience of infertility and reproductive loss really is. For those who suffer, it's an isolating situation. Nobody really understands what it's like unless they've been through it. And nobody really talks about it.

In our own counseling training programs, we remember the debate about whether we could truly help clients if we had never experienced what they had, if we'd not been there, done that. Can you effectively work with an addict if you've never faced addiction? Can you successfully help someone walk through a divorce if your own marriage experience is happily ever after? Can you really help another person heal from depression if you've never endured and overcome deep despair? Some say yes. They say with genuineness and empathy and unconditional positive regard, along with some education and tried and true strategies, you can. Some say no. Those on this side of the debate say you can be of some help, but you will never be as effective if you don't know firsthand the unique pain and suffering of the client.

For helping professionals working with infertility, we wonder if the same debate applies. On one hand, you can show empathy. You can show compassion. You can walk the path of healing with a client, a supervisee, or a student. On the other hand, if you've never been through it, you'll never know the depth of the hurt. The pain. The suffering. The grief. The isolation. And that is what sufferers really need you to know. How much infertility hurts. And how much they need someone to listen. And how much they need someone to care.

DOI: 10.4324/9781003336402-3

And how much they need hope. And how much they need healing. That is the reason for this book. For all those who so desperately want to have a baby and can't ... let's talk about why it really is such a big deal.

Current estimates suggest that 48 million couples and 186 million individuals live with infertility globally. That's about 15% of the population (World Health Organization, 2020) or around one in eight people. In the United States alone, 19% of heterosexual women between the ages of 15–49 cannot get pregnant after a year of trying, and 26% cannot get pregnant or carry a pregnancy to term (Centers for Disease Control, n.d.). Yet despite these numbers of epidemic proportions, infertility is infrequently in the spotlight.

Many conditions have designated awareness months. If you conduct a quick online search using the term "health awareness months," you'll find several websites listing all the health-related issues we observe. Here are just a few. January raises awareness for glaucoma. February has the heart. March brings attention to brain injury. Even irritable bowel syndrome is honored with its own month in April. Societally, we remember and offer support to millions of sufferers of a variety of conditions. Many even have their own movements that are recognized by campaigns and colored ribbons. This isn't the case for infertility.

While infertility is not a widely discussed issue, some advocates have endeavored to make it more well-known. Many thanks to RESOLVE (The National Infertility Association), which has designated one week each April as National Infertility Awareness Week (RESOLVE, n.d.). And now, some proponents have begun recognizing World Infertility Awareness Month in June. While you may not hear much about it, knowledge of the condition is growing. Even celebrities are speaking out about their own struggles. Those who have publicly discussed these challenges include Anne Hathaway, Michelle Obama, Kim Kardashian, Mark Zuckerberg, and Hugh Jackman. Still, much of the struggle with infertility continues to be inward, personal, and silent. People don't talk about it. It's painful. It's stigmatizing. It's isolating.

WHAT CAN HELPING PROFESSIONALS DO?

Healthcare providers are the main source of treating this biological issue. However, infertility impacts individuals far beyond the physical realm. Infertility is a complex, multifaceted crisis that impacts sufferers biologically, psychologically, and socially. While some seek professional counseling to assist with the physical, emotional, and relational issues related to infertility, many do not. Reasons could include stigma, finances, lack of access to a mental health professional, or maybe not even realizing they need help. And although a wide range of conferences, webinars, and trainings are available for helping professionals to learn more about their craft, instruction and education infrequently focus on infertility. As a result, many may lack the experience, knowledge, or skills needed to assist this population with the healing process.

Since one in eight individuals suffer from infertility, there's a good chance at some point in your career you will encounter clients, supervisees, students, or friends and family members of those who battle infertility and reproductive loss as well as the accompanying grief and sorrow related to the condition. You may be wondering how you can help, especially if you don't know much about it. Maybe you're a counselor working with a client who, while in session, breaks down in tears when describing years of negative pregnancy tests. How can you truly understand her experience if your pregnancy tests were always positive? Maybe you're a supervisor working with a counselor-in-training who is struggling with grief related to having multiple miscarriages. How can you provide quality supervision when she describes feelings of countertransference when working with a pregnant client? Maybe you're a counselor educator who has a student who has struggled. How can you provide support as they work through chronic sorrow associated with the loss of a personal dream while at the same time working through the rigor of pursuing a professional dream? This book aims to be a guide to help with all these situations whether you, the professional, have experienced infertility or not.

And let's face it. If you're reading this book, statistically, chances are some of you have experienced infertility and/or reproductive loss. How do you handle it when it comes up in a session? In class? Or with a supervisee? How can you effectively help others when they stir up emotions related to your own personal struggles? And if you've never experienced infertility, how can you effectively help them if you've never dealt with the issues they're facing? This book will give you the knowledge and the tools to answer these questions.

We divided this book into three parts. In the first section, we explore the biopsychosocial crisis of infertility and the ways in which the condition affects individuals biologically, psychologically, and socially. In the second section, we address the experience of those who suffer, moving beyond just women to include men, other partners, extended family members, and members of diverse populations. In the third and final section, we focus on practical tools, strategies, and suggestions for assisting others, and maybe even yourself, with the journey of infertility and reproductive loss.

We use the metaphor of the literary format of the Hero's Journey because those who suffer have much in common with some of our favorite well-known heroes. Consider Frodo Baggins, Harry Potter, Luke Skywalker, and Dorothy from The Wizard of Oz. Each goes on an adventure (sometimes not of their own choosing), is challenged with a decisive crisis, and, after the resolution of the crisis, returns transformed. The infertility journey certainly parallels these phases. It is an adventure filled with many twists and turns. It involves crises that must be decisively overcome. And no matter what the outcome, the sufferer is transformed as part of the process. And let's face it. A hero is someone who is admired or idealized for courage, outstanding achievements, or noble qualities. We so admire your clients, supervisees, students, and even you, for the courage you have to help others on the journey of infertility … and for maybe even facing it yourself. This book is for you.

THE HERO'S JOURNEY

Some heroes' stories, like Frodo and Dorothy, are known around the world. Some stories are more personal and hit closer to home such as the story of the quintessential little girl. Maybe her story is similar to yours. Let's start at the very beginning.

Once upon a time in a land not so far away, a beautiful baby girl is born. Her delighted parents name her Jane. They found out several months ago she was going to be a girl, so they painted the nursery pink and bought dresses and bows for her to wear. And what kinds of toys did they buy for Jane? Dolls. Lots and lots of dolls. From a young age, Jane loved playing with them. She rocked them and changed them and combed their hair. She fed them and strolled them and sang lullabies to them as they went to sleep. And Jane dreamed about the day she would have real live babies of her own. She watched Disney movies and dreamed of Prince Charming and finding happily ever after. Then Jane grew up. She finished school. She started a career. She did find Prince Charming, and they began building their future. When they bought a house, they made sure it had four bedrooms … one for them and three for the little ones they planned to have one day.

But that day never came.

When considering the plight of infertility and reproductive loss, it is imperative to remember that no two stories are the same. While the story of little Jane may be familiar to some, it's not all-encompassing. Not all individuals have experienced traditional gender-role stereotyping. Not all dream of finding Prince Charming. Not all want the house with the white picket fence. But even though the stories vary, infertility can strike them all. Consider these scenarios.

- Luna, age 29, has suffered from five miscarriages within the last two years. She and her partner seek the help of a reproductive endocrinologist who diagnoses a blood clotting disorder. Shortly after beginning treatment, she conceives and gives birth to a baby boy. However, she continues to experience depression related to her losses.
- Rhonda, age 35, was diagnosed with endometriosis at the age of 19. After twelve years of grueling infertility treatments including endometrial surgery and in vitro fertilization, she has given up hope. Now she deals with the chronic sorrow that she'll never have children of her own.

- Acacia, age 34, has one child. She's not getting any younger, so she begins working on Baby #2. She and her spouse are unable to pay for the high cost of infertility treatments, so after six years of trying the natural way, she gives up hope. She grieves the loss of her dream of having a house full of children and siblings for her daughter. But she also experiences disenfranchised grief because her family does not acknowledge her pain. None of them ask how she's doing. None has ever said, "I'm sorry you're going through a hard time." This lack of support leads Acacia to wonder if they care at all, and her grief is complicated by secondary loss.
- Liam, age 42, and his wife long for a child of their own. After four years of trying for a baby, they seek professional help. Following a battery of tests, the physician discovers Liam's sperm count is extremely low. He feels like a failure as a husband and grieves the loss of his manhood. He also worries his wife will view him differently. The couple visits a sperm bank, and his wife is artificially inseminated. She is excited about the process, but he is hesitant and worries if he can love a child that isn't biologically his.

These stories are just the beginning. There are millions of others worldwide with similar themes but with very different characters, very different plot twists, and very different endings. These stories are part of the Hero's Journey, the twists and turns, the ups and downs, and the ins and outs of the road called infertility … the quest that leaves no one unchanged.

CONCLUSION

The Hero's Journey is intense and wrought with difficulty, trouble, and danger. Just like heroes from other stories, those experiencing infertility and reproductive loss will encounter intense difficulties, troubles, and even dangers related to their overall health and well-being. The biopsychosocial model explores the association between biological, psychological, and social factors related to a variety of topics ranging from human development to health and disease. In the next three chapters, we explore this biopsychosocial crisis to help you better understand the interconnection between physical, mental, and relational challenges faced by those suffering from infertility. We also address the ways in which these challenges negatively impact overall health and well-being. Our hope is that you will gain insight into how complex the issue really is and how it impacts every part of a person's life. May you gain empathy and understanding for those who are affected. And if one of those affected is you, may this book be a part of your own healing journey. Because infertility is such a big deal. And you are our hero.

REFERENCES

Centers for Disease Control (n.d.). *Infertility*. Retrieved October 7, 2022, from https://www.cdc.gov/reproductivehealth/infertility/

RESOLVE (n.d.). *National Infertility Awareness Week*. Retrieved October 7, 2022, from https://resolve.org/events/national-infertility-awareness-week/

World Health Organization (2020, September 14). *Infertility*. https://www.who.int/news-room/fact-sheets/detail/infertility

CHAPTER TWO

Biological Impacts of Infertility

My Body Betrayed Me

My body betrayed me.

For many who experience infertility, this is a common sentiment. Let's return to the analogy of the Hero's Journey and begin with our female hero. She lives a somewhat normal existence. She works. She plays. She dreams. She plans. She fulfills her duties and obligations. She satisfies her roles and responsibilities. She goes about her daily business without much distraction or trouble.

And then, something happens.

The call to adventure for most heroes is a loss of some kind. For the hero in the story of infertility, the call is often triggered by a loss of health … more specifically, her reproductive health. She goes from a relatively well-functioning body to one defined by a medical diagnosis. Her body doesn't work like it's supposed to. Something that seems to happen so easily for others is a struggle for her. This biological problem takes the hero on a journey she never wanted or thought she would have.

Many people wrongly assume the journey to having a baby is linear. You decide to have a baby. You get pregnant. You give birth. You live happily ever after. However, for those suffering from infertility and reproductive loss, the journey is never that easy. Instead, the road is filled with ups, downs, twists, and turns. Sometimes it's bumpy. Sometimes it's rocky. And sometimes the ending isn't happy. And for many, the loss of reproductive health is a catalyst for so many other losses. In the remainder of this chapter, we explore the diagnosis of infertility and the biological crisis it creates. This is the first step in the call to adventure.

Warning to all readers. This chapter can get technical. If you currently work as a helping professional or are in the process of becoming one, chances are the hard sciences were not your favorite subjects in school. Why? You probably consider yourself a people person. You possess natural abilities when it comes to interpersonal and intrapersonal skills. Friends and family members come to you for advice. You can't get enough of psychology and what makes people tick. The amoeba and cytoplasm, on the other hand? Not so much. We realize some of you may have loved all things biology, and this chapter may be your cup of tea. But for the rest, you may already have thoughts of skipping it. We would ask you to please not pass it by.

We want you to know this information is so very important to have in working with those suffering from infertility and reproductive loss. Why? Sufferers need someone to empathize with them, and, in order to do that, you need a little insight into their experiences. Physicians are often the first line of treatment when it comes to infertility. And while some are extremely under-standing and helpful, many are so focused on the science of conception that they neglect the heartfelt empathy that could really benefit patients during the grueling process of diagnosis and treatment.

So, if, and when, you work with those suffering from infertility, you'll be a step ahead of the game if you know a little about what they're up against. Take it from firsthand experience. Sometimes you just want someone to listen. To understand. To hurt with you. And part of understanding and empathizing and hurting together stems from the knowledge of the biological aspects of infertility and reproductive loss. We'll try to not bog you down with too many technical terms, so you may want to explore these issues more in-depth from other sources. But our hope is this information will serve as a solid foundation for becoming more aware of the physical challenges associated with infertility. We have also created a glossary of terms at the end of this book for quick reference. Let's get started.

According to The American College of Obstetricians and Gynecologists (2019), a diagnosis of infertility is established when pregnancy is not achieved within one year of unprotected intercourse or one year of therapeutic donor insemination. The caveat is the one-year rule applies only if a woman is younger than 35 years of age. For those over 35, the time frame for conception to occur is only six months because of the need for earlier intervention due to age.

There are two main types of infertility. Primary infertility occurs when a couple has never conceived, and secondary infertility is diagnosed when people have achieved pregnancy at least once but then are unable to con-ceive again (World Health Organization, 2020). Those suffering from infertility should schedule an appointment with a reproductive endocrinologist who is a gynecologist with specialized training in both male and female infertility issues as well as recurrent pregnancy loss (Centers for Disease Control, n.d.-a). The reproductive endocrinologist can assess, diagnose, and treat infertility issues. You'll read more about that later. For now, let's continue our discussion of reproductive challenges with the process of conception.

The process of natural conception begins when an egg is released from a woman's ovary and travels down the fallopian tubes. As it travels, sperm swim up through the vagina and into the uterus to join with the egg. The fertilized egg continues its journey down the fallopian tubes where it implants, or attaches, to the lining of the uterus. At this point, the body produces hormones that prevent the shedding of the lining of the uterus. The uterus maintains its lining, and the woman misses her period. This is often the first indication of pregnancy (Cleveland Clinic, n.d.-c). It sounds like an uncomplicated process. And for most people, it usually is. But for those suffering from infertility, conception is a sizable challenge. See Figure 2.1 for a diagram of human fertilization.

To treat infertility, reproductive endocrinologists must first determine why conception is not occurring. In about one-third of cases, infertility is due to female factors and about one-third is due to male factors. The final one-third of cases are due to unexplained causes or a combination of factors (National Institute of Child Health and Human Development, n.d.). We should also point out that people who are single or in same-sex relationships may face unique challenges when it comes to treating infertility because of the barriers they already face to achieve natural conception. This barrier, compounded with an infertility diagnosis, may be particularly difficult for them.

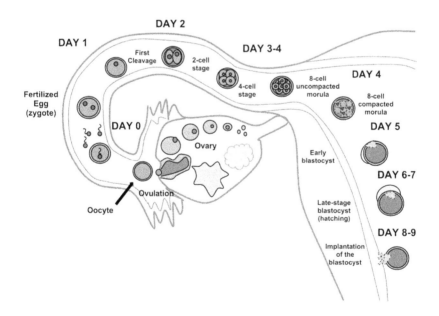

FIGURE 2.1 The Process of Fertilization

Source: https://commons.wikimedia.org/w/index.php?curid=19679961#file

How do physicians know where to start? The initial diagnosis usually includes a routine medical examination and exploration of medical history. Questions related to medical history may include the use of medications, any past pregnancies, environmental risk factors such as pollution, industrial chemicals, and radiation, known illnesses, lifestyle factors like drug and alcohol use, family medical history, and sexual history, including any sexually transmitted infections. The physician also conducts a thorough physical examination to assess overall health and wellness such as thyroid health which can be an indicator of a potential problem. In addition, a gynecological exam consisting of a pelvic exam and pap smear will assess reproductive health. Patients answer questions related to menstrual cycles, irregularities, abnormal bleeding, discharges, and any pelvic pain (The American College of Obstetricians and Gynecologists, 2019).

Some physicians pursue additional testing including lab tests, imaging tests, or other procedures to evaluate fertility. Lab tests may include those for hormones, thyroid function, and egg supply. Imaging tests and procedures include transvaginal ultrasound, sonohysterography, hysterosalpingography, hysteroscopy, and laparoscopy. A transvaginal ultrasound is a procedure that examines organs such as the bladder, uterus, vagina, and fallopian tubes. Sound waves bounce off organs inside the pelvis from an instrument that has been inserted into the vagina (National Cancer Institute, n.d.-b). It may determine antral follicle count, which provides valuable information about ovarian reserve and will help predict response to medications that stimulate the ovaries. The sonohysterogram and hysterosalpingogram involve injecting fluid into the uterus and fallopian tubes to check for blockages. In rare instances, hysteroscopy and laparoscopy may be performed. These minimally invasive procedures investigate potential abnormalities or irregularities with the reproductive organs.

And let's not forget the men. Semen analysis can determine any problems with sperm count, shape, and/or movement. To produce a semen sample, men must either masturbate, have sex with a condom, use the withdrawal method prior to ejaculation, or ejaculate via electrical stimulation (Johnson, 2017). Blood tests can measure reproductive hormones, and scrotal ultrasound can assess problems in the testicles (The American College of Obstetricians and Gynecologists, 2020) which can negatively impact male fertility.

Whew! Are we having fun yet? Our heads were spinning as we learned about these things on our own journeys, so we figure yours are, too. But this is only the beginning. Now take a moment and put yourself in the shoes of the person going through the process. The whirlwind of appointments, new terminology, and testing procedures along with the uncertainty of the outcome is a crisis in itself, not to mention the challenge of admitting something is wrong, the fears of moving from a regular physician to a specialist, the discomfort, pain, and embarrassment of invasive procedures, and the changes to an intimate part of a partner relationship. Some people at this point may already begin to experience grief. Yet most continue to have hope, believing if they can find the cause, they can then move forward with a treatment plan which may resolve the issue and result in a child.

CAUSES OF INFERTILITY

There are numerous causes of infertility. Sometimes the causes are related to issues present from birth. Sometimes problems occur later in life, and these problems can result from female issues, male issues, or a combination of both. Unfortunately, in many cases, the cause remains unknown. Here's a deeper look at some possible causes of infertility.

In females, many factors can impact how easily a woman ovulates, gets pregnant, or gives birth to a child. These factors can include maternal age, ovulation disorders, fallopian tube damage or blockage, uterine or cervical abnormalities, endometriosis, pelvic adhesions, cancer and its treatment, chronic diseases, environmental factors, and sexually transmitted infections. In males, causes are mostly related to abnormal sperm production or function, problems with the delivery of sperm, overexposure to certain environmental factors, and damage related to cancer and its treatment. Other risk factors can affect both males and females. These include age, tobacco use, alcohol use, being either overweight or underweight, disordered eating, and excessive exercise issues. Let's begin with female factors.

Female Factors

About one-third of infertility cases are due to female factors (National Institute of Child Health and Human Development, n.d.) and are typically attributed to problems with the ovaries, fallopian tubes, uterus, and cervix. Ovulation disorders are caused by problems with the regulation of reproductive hormones which affect egg production and release and are some of the most common causes of infertility in women (Centers for Disease Control, n.d.-a). Culprits include dysfunction of the pituitary gland or hypothalamus, premature ovarian insufficiency (the ovaries stop working normally before the age of 40), diminished ovarian reserve (decreased number of eggs available), polycystic ovarian syndrome (a hormonal disorder causing enlarged ovaries with small cysts on the outer edges), cessation of ovulation (due to stress, disordered eating, or intense exercise), and menopause (Centers for Disease Control, n.d.-a).

Another common source of problems is fallopian tube damage or blockage. This is often caused by inflammation of the fallopian tubes. Blockage or damage contributes to infertility because the fallopian tubes are typically where sperm fertilize the egg. If the tubes are blocked or damaged, the sperm and/or fertilized egg may not travel smoothly. Damage or blockage can result from a ruptured appendix, pelvic infection, endometriosis, sexually transmitted infections, and previous pelvic surgeries (Centers for Disease Control, n.d.-a).

The uterus and cervix also impact fertility. Problems with a woman's uterus or cervix can be caused by a variety of factors. These include fibroids, adhesions, polyps, abnormal tissue growth in the uterine wall, congenital issues, and prior surgeries or procedures (Centers for Disease Control, n.d.-a). In addition, certain types of cervical mucus may impact the movement of sperm, and sometimes antibodies in the mucus kill sperm or prevent them from moving normally (Rebar, 2020). The primary symptom is usually the inability to conceive, although many women with uterine abnormalities may also experience recurrent miscarriages. See Figure 2.2 for a diagram of the female reproductive organs.

Another contributing factor is certain types of cancer, especially reproductive cancer and its treatment which can impair the ability to conceive. This is especially true when treatment involves surgical procedures including the removal of tumors near reproductive organs or the removal of reproductive organs themselves. In addition, other treatments such as radiation, chemotherapy, and hormone therapy can negatively affect fertility (National Cancer Institute, n.d.-a).

Finally, chronic diseases, environmental factors, and maternal age can contribute to female infertility. Chronic diseases impacting fertility include hypertension, lupus, diabetes, arthritis, and asthma (Johns Hopkins Medicine, n.d.). Environmental factors consist of exposure to hazardous materials such as alcohol and drug use, toxins in the workplace, and other contaminants; and

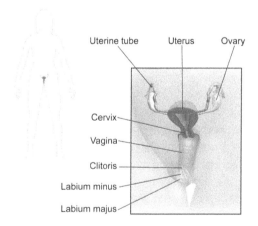

FIGURE 2.2 The Female Reproductive System

Source: Blausen.com staff (2014). "Medical gallery of Blausen Medical 2014". WikiJournal of Medicine 1 (2). DOI: 10.15347/wjm/2014.010. ISSN 2002-4436.

when considering maternal age, women in their late 30s and older are less fertile than women in their 20s (Johns Hopkins Medicine, n.d.).

Male Factors

About one-third of infertility problems are attributed to male factors (National Institute of Child Health and Human Development, n.d.). These typically involve problems with the sperm or testicles. Abnormal sperm production or function is a common cause of male factor infertility. Many physicians will conduct a semen analysis to assess the number of sperm (concentration), their movement (motility), and their shape (morphology) (Centers for Disease Control, n.d.-a). Sperm with head or tail defects may be unable to reach or penetrate the egg (Helo, 2022). Sometimes no sperm are produced at all. This is called azoospermia (Cleveland Clinic, n.d.-a).

When it comes to the testicles, a diagnosis of varicocele is one of the most common causes of male infertility. It involves a swelling of the veins in the testicles that may impact sperm quality and quantity (Centers for Disease Control, n.d.-a). Problems with the delivery of sperm from the testicles can also interfere with conception. Hormonal problems, trauma to the testes, and genetic abnormalities could also play a part (Centers for Disease Control, n.d.-a). Heavy drug or alcohol use, cancer treatment (including chemotherapy, radiation, and surgery), and medical conditions such as diabetes and cystic fibrosis can be a culprit, too (Centers for Disease Control (n.d.-a). See Figure 2.3 for a diagram of the male reproductive organs.

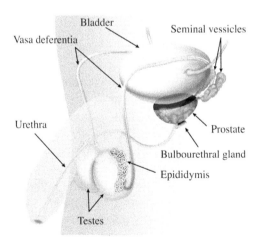

FIGURE 2.3 The Male Reproductive System

Source: https://commons.wikimedia.org/wiki/File:Sperm_release_pathway.svg

Unexplained Infertility

So far, we've discussed both male and female factors that can cause infertility. In the final one-third of infertility cases, no cause is identified (National Institute of Child Health and Human Development, n.d.). When no cause is determined, infertility is described as unexplained (Centers for Disease Control, n.d.-a). Unexplained infertility is most likely due to poor egg or sperm quality or with problems with the uterus or fallopian tubes. These problems just weren't identifiable during normal fertility testing. This situation can be extremely frustrating for individuals because they know there is a problem but are unable to pinpoint what it is. This makes it difficult to move forward with a distinct treatment plan tailored to the individual's needs.

REPRODUCTIVE LOSS

In the first part of this chapter, we discussed the process of conception, explored different types of infertility testing, and described various causes for infertility. Next, let's spend some time focusing on another type of challenge: reproductive loss. For some individuals and couples, infertility is the crisis that serves as the catalyst for the Hero's Journey. For some, however, the inability to conceive is not a crisis at all. Instead, their journey includes the experience of reproductive loss. These types of losses include chemical and ectopic pregnancy, miscarriage, recurrent pregnancy loss, stillbirth, abortion, premature birth, early infant death, special needs diagnosis, and sterilization.

Chemical and Ectopic Pregnancy

A typical pregnancy lasts 40 weeks. A chemical pregnancy is defined as a pregnancy that ends before the fifth week; it's a type of miscarriage, but there are often no symptoms because although an embryo forms and may even implant, it then stops developing (Cleveland Clinic, n.d.-b). On the other hand, an ectopic pregnancy occurs when implantation of the fertilized egg takes place outside the uterus. If left to grow, it may damage other organs and result in life-threatening loss of blood for the mother. Symptoms include pelvic pain and vaginal bleeding. In the early stages of pregnancy, medication may be the only treatment needed to end the pregnancy. In later stages, surgery is required (The American College of Obstetricians and Gynecologists, 2018).

Miscarriage

Miscarriage, sometimes called spontaneous abortion, is defined as the spontaneous loss of a pregnancy before the 20th week (Dugas & Slane, 2022). The experience can be both physically and emotionally painful. Miscarriage is the most common type of pregnancy loss, and it often occurs because the fetus isn't developing normally. This is usually due to chromosomal issues or maternal health conditions such as problems with the uterus, cervix, hormones, infections, uncontrolled diabetes, and thyroid disease (Mayo Clinic, 2021b). Some people experience multiple miscarriages. This is referred to as recurrent pregnancy loss and is diagnosed when two or more miscarriages have occurred (The American College of Obstetricians and Gynecologists, 2016). The risk of miscarriage increases with the number of previous pregnancy losses but is typically less than 50%. Reproductive specialists can evaluate and treat these issues in hopes of achieving a full-term pregnancy, but in more than one-half of patients with recurrent pregnancy loss, the cause is unexplained (The American College of Obstetricians and Gynecologists, 2016).

Stillbirth

Stillbirth is the death or loss of a baby before or during delivery. While miscarriage occurs prior to the 20th week of pregnancy, stillbirth is defined as a loss of a baby at or after the 20th week (Centers for Disease Control, n.d.-b). An early stillbirth occurs between 20 and 27 weeks, a late stillbirth occurs between 28 and 36 weeks, and a term stillbirth occurs between 37 or more weeks of pregnancy. About 24,000 babies are stillborn in the United States each year, and in about one-third of these cases, the reasons are unexplained. The other two-thirds may be caused by problems with the placenta or umbilical cord, infections, birth defects, high blood pressure, or poor lifestyle choices. In addition, an unexplained stillbirth is more likely to occur the farther along a woman is in her pregnancy (Centers for Disease Control, n.d.-b).

Abortion

An abortion ends a pregnancy with medical intervention. It uses medication or surgical procedures to remove the embryo or fetus and placenta from the uterus (Lee & Kahn, 2021). Individuals who have abortions can also experience feelings of grief and loss, even if the abortion is elective. Several types of abortion procedures exist including medical abortion, vacuum aspiration, dilation and evacuation, prostaglandin abortion, and late-term abortion. Medical abortion occurs when medications are used to end a pregnancy of approximately 10 weeks or less. Vacuum aspiration is a surgical technique used during the first trimester. Dilation and evacuation (D and E) are used for pregnancy termination between 13 and 21 weeks. Second-trimester pregnancies can be terminated with prostaglandins, which are hormones causing uterine contractions which lead to the delivery of the fetus and placenta. And late-term abortions, or intact dilation and extraction, are performed between 20 and 24 weeks (Lee & Kahn, 2021). First-trimester abortion does not seem to have a significant effect on future fertility or pregnancy. However, women who have abortions later in their pregnancies may experience complications when trying to conceive again later in life. In this case, the inability to conceive coupled with potential feelings of self-blame and guilt related to previous abortions may intensify the individual's experience of grief and loss.

Premature Birth and Early Infant Death

Premature birth occurs when a baby is born prior to the 37th week of pregnancy (Mayo Clinic, 2021a). Some risk factors for preterm birth include having a previous preterm birth, multiple pregnancies, infections, chronic conditions, or being pregnant with multiples. Complications for the newborn include immature lungs, poor feeding, slow weight gain, and difficulty regulating body temperature. Babies may need intense nursery care, medications, or sometimes surgery (Mayo Clinic, 2021a). Sometimes premature babies, or even full-term babies, do not survive. Early infant death, or neonatal death, occurs when a baby dies within the first 28 days of life. The most common causes are premature birth, low birth weight, and birth defects (March of Dimes, n.d.-b).

JENNIFER'S STORY

After many years of undergoing infertility treatments, my husband and I finally got the news that we were pregnant ... with twins! The first trimester of my pregnancy and most of the 2nd trimester were relatively uneventful and went as expected. The boys measured smaller than anticipated, but that was expected for twins. I went in for my 28-week checkup and was scheduled to have my glucose test done. We went to have the ultrasound first, as usual, but the technician was not very forthcoming with information during the scan and took many more images than in previous appointments. At the time we didn't think too far into things as we could see both babies and both were showing lots of movement. After a very long wait in the doctor's office, we were finally visited by the OB who informed us that I would be admitted to the hospital within the hour. I was exhibiting signs of preeclampsia, and blood flow going to both boys was less than it should have been. I was only in the hospital for five days, with the boys just barely at 29 weeks, when the decision was made to do the c-section. Blood flow to Christopher had been totally compromised. With preeclampsia, the umbilical vessels can narrow, which they did, and this caused blood to actually be taken from Christopher's body instead of him taking blood from mine. Blood flow to Trevor had been lessened as well, so he was at risk, too. I had already been injected with steroids to encourage maturity of the boys' lungs, but they were still so small. Christopher was 1 lb. 10 oz, and Trevor was 2 lb. 3 oz, and both were less than a foot in length. Both needed to go to the NICU, and both needed to be on oxygen right away as their lungs were not ready to function on their own. Doctors determined that both needed surfactant applied to their lungs within their first 24 hours to help oxygenation be more efficient. Trevor did well with this, but Christopher did not. Christopher suffered a massive lung hemorrhage and needed many blood transfusions and many, many prayers. Doctors could not predict Christopher's outcome, and he was not even a day old at this point. Once they were able to suction out the blood, Christopher was placed on an oscillator for breathing to help his lungs recover. With each passing day, the boys were growing stronger, but issues were still present. Their brains would forget to breathe and forget to tell their heart to beat – all prematurity complications, but terrifying for us. After spending 79 days in the NICU, eventually both were able to finally get off breathing support and feeding support. In their first year home, they were still seeing many specialists to track their progress as many complications are seen with premature children. By the end of their second year, they had been cleared from all their specialists and thankfully were developing as expected. Even to this day, the major lasting effects from their prematurity primarily have to do with their lungs. Both have reactive airway disease – which basically means that their lungs remain incredibly sensitive to irritants and getting infections.

My husband and I both would completely agree that we now carry posttraumatic stress disorder from our experiences with the boys. The thought of being able to bring a full size baby home directly after birth will never fully have a place in our minds. I was not even able to hold either of the boys until they were already a week old, and then it was incredibly brief. The boys were surrounded in the NICU by many other babies - at this time all in an open room – which exposed us to other, often more severe cases and much infant death. We would go to see our boys in the NICU, and it would often be temporarily closed to visitors due to a loss from one of the families. When I think back to bottle feeding the boys with my pumped breastmilk, I think about how tiny the volumes of milk were and how as soon as they began sucking the bottle they would forget to breathe and their heart would stop, so we were constantly on edge then as well. The thought of bringing them home was daunting … what if they stopped breathing then, too? Thankfully, the wonderful nurses trained us well as to how to respond, and those days seem like forever ago. To say that we are still overly cautious, even now that they are six years, old is an understatement. As the boys slowly build their immunity, we are trying our best to be less overprotective, but that is beyond difficult when you can still see images of those times in the NICU when things were very different and very, very scary.

Birth of Special Needs Children

We consider the birth of a special needs child another type of reproductive loss. This is not to undervalue those of the disability community or undermine their unique circumstances. Our aim here is only to recognize the grief experienced by parents that often accompanies a special needs diagnosis. The diagnosis may have been made either prior to the birth or after the birth, but feelings of grief can still occur the way they do with other types of loss. About three percent of babies are born with birth defects each year in the United States (March of Dimes, n.d.-a). While giving birth is typically a joyous occasion, a sense of grief can overshadow the joy. The birth of an infant with a disability may require additional support from healthcare professionals during and after the birthing process. Additionally, news of the diagnosis can bring about a grief reaction including sadness and despair at the loss of a dream for the perfect baby and a "normal" future.

Sterilization

Finally, we explore sterilization. Sterilization is a permanent form of birth control. For women, sterilization is called tubal or female sterilization and can occur in two ways. First, through a minor surgical procedure, a section of both fallopian tubes or the entire tubes themselves are removed. Second, and less commonly, clips are used to close off the fallopian tubes. These procedures prevent the egg from traveling down the tubes and the sperm from reaching the egg. For men, sterilization is called vasectomy. The procedure involves tying, cutting, clipping, or sealing the tube that carries sperm from the testicles. This prevents a woman's egg from being fertilized (The American College of Obstetricians and Gynecologists, 2022). Sterilization is permanent birth control. If someone who is sterilized changes their mind, they can attempt surgery to reverse it unless the entire fallopian tube was removed. In this instance, in vitro fertilization would be the only option to achieve a pregnancy. These procedures are not always successful which may trigger feelings of grief-related reproductive loss. Sometimes sterilization may have occurred with a previous partner. This can further complicate the grieving process.

TREATMENT

No matter the cause of infertility or the type of reproductive loss experienced, the course of action will depend on the problem. Some will attempt various types of treatment in order to conceive. However, some choose not to pursue medical intervention and instead seek alternative routes to parenthood. We discuss these alternatives in Chapter 9. For now, we delve into treatments for infertility which consist of three main types: medications, surgical procedures, and assisted conception.

Medications

Medications for infertility can treat both women and men. For women, they assist with ovulation problems. Some encourage the monthly release of an egg in those who do not ovulate regularly or at all, and others can help stimulate ovulation. Medications for men may also improve fertility by increasing testosterone levels. However, some of these medications may cause side effects such as headaches, hot flashes, nausea, and vomiting. They may also trigger other issues including mood swings and an increased risk of multiples (American Pregnancy Association, n.d.).

Surgical Procedures

A variety of surgical procedures exist that can treat infertility. For women, fallopian tube surgery can repair blocked or scarred fallopian tubes. Surgery may also be used to identify and correct polyps, endometriosis, fibroids, and other growths (NYU Langone Health, n.d.-a). In men, surgery may help improve sperm production, correct blockages that prevent sperm from being ejaculated properly, or can reverse vasectomy. In addition, sperm can be surgically extracted in cases of obstruction, missing vas deferens (the tube that drains sperm from the testicle), and vasectomy or failed vasectomy reversal (NYU Langone Health, n.d.-b).

Assisted Conception

Last, we focus on assisted conception. Sometimes physicians perform procedures to assist with conception. Two examples are ovulation induction (OI) and intrauterine insemination (IUI). With ovulation induction, fertility medications are used to stimulate egg production in the ovaries; intrauterine insemination can be used in conjunction with ovulation induction and involves placing sperm directly into the uterus with a small catheter (Yale Medicine, n.d.).

Other forms of assisted conception are called Assisted Reproductive Technologies (ART). Examples include in vitro fertilization (IVF), zygote intrafallopian transfer (ZIFT), and gamete intrafallopian transfer (GIFT) (Society for Assisted Reproductive Technology, n.d.). In vitro fertilization involves combining sperm and eggs in a laboratory and then placing the embryos in the uterus (Mitchell & Christianson, 2021). With zygote intrafallopian transfer, the fertilized eggs are introduced into the fallopian tubes. And with gamete intrafallopian transfer, the sperm and eggs are mixed together and inserted in the fallopian tubes in hopes fertilization of the egg will occur (Kaiser Permanente, 2020). Zygote intrafallopian transfer and gamete intrafallopian transfer are closer to natural conception than in vitro fertilization; however, they require surgical procedures that in vitro fertilization does not. Therefore, in vitro fertilization is the preferred choice for most clinics and is used 98% of the time (Choe et al., 2022). These procedures can be very costly and often wreak havoc on a woman's body from the medications that impact hormones and the invasive procedures to assess various stages of egg production, release, and retrieval. Still, this is a popular course of action for many who cannot conceive through other methods.

Other types of assisted conception include egg donation, sperm donation, embryo donation, or surrogacy. How can these options help? Perhaps a couple is unable to provide their own eggs, sperm, or embryos due to medical issues such as no or low-quality sperm and eggs. Some may not want to risk passing down genetic disorders (American Society for Reproductive Medicine, n.d.). These options can assist individuals and couples as they pursue the path to parenthood. Let's explore how these alternatives work.

With egg or sperm donation, the process is similar to in vitro fertilization. Donated eggs are combined with a partner's sperm or donated sperm are combined with a partner's eggs and then the embryos are placed in the uterus (UNC Fertility, n.d.). Embryo donation is another form of treatment in which individuals adopt embryos that have been frozen by other people as part of their in vitro fertilization process, but those people decided not to use them. This thawing and transfer of frozen embryos is called frozen embryo transfer, or FET (Shah, 2020).

Finally, some people choose surrogacy. This is a method of assisted conception where couples work with a gestational surrogate who will carry and care for their baby until birth (UNC Fertility, n.d.). Those who choose surrogacy can use embryos made up of their own eggs and sperm, embryos made of one partner's egg or sperm combined with a donor's egg or sperm, or they may adopt embryos that are implanted in the surrogate.

GRIEVING BIOLOGICAL LOSSES

We've combed through multiple layers contributing to the biological crisis of infertility. These include testing, diagnosis, and treatment, as well as many types of reproductive loss. Now, with a clearer understanding of the biological crisis, we'd like to note that throughout this entire process, it is completely normal and extremely common for people to experience grief at many different levels. Grief is a psychological issue we explore extensively in Chapter 3. However, it's important to point out that many of our heroes will grieve biological losses as part of their journey. Here are a few examples.

- A teenager may grieve a loss of health when she gets a diagnosis of polycystic ovarian syndrome and a warning from her doctor that pregnancy may not come easily.
- A woman may grieve the loss of a dream she had for her body to experience pregnancy and childbirth when she starts her period month after month, year after year, without conceiving.
- A couple may experience loss of life when their countless pregnancies result in multiple miscarriages.

It is crucial that you are aware of these losses as you explore clients' unique stories as well as the grief associated with them. This may become even more vital if pregnancy, birth, and/or parenthood are never achieved.

CONCLUSION

You made it! We hope that as a result of reading this chapter, you have a better understanding of the complex and complicated biological circumstances unique to each individual who experiences infertility and/or seeks medical intervention to treat it. You may have already been familiar with some of this content, but if not, you're practically an expert now. Infertility brings about a biological crisis of overwhelming proportions that changes people's lives … and trajectories … forever. In your work with these individuals, you must open your hearts and open your minds. Listen. Empathize. Question. Care. They need you to understand what they're experiencing, and they need you to sit with them through the pain. You may be the only one who does. Your work becomes even more crucial as the biological crisis sets the stage for a complex series of reactions that can also impact mental and relational well-being. We'll end the discussion of the biological crisis here and, in the next chapter, explore the psychological crisis of infertility.

REFERENCES

American Pregnancy Association (n.d.). *Fertility medications*. Retrieved September 24, 2022, from https://americanpregnancy.org/getting-pregnant/fertility-medications/

American Society for Reproductive Medicine (n.d.). *Gamete (eggs and sperm) and embryo donation*. Retrieved September 24, 2022, from https://www. reproductivefacts.org/news-and-publications/patient-fact-sheets-and-booklets/documents/fact-sheets-and-info-booklets/gamete-eggs-and-sperm-and-embryo-donation/#:~:text=Some%20people%20use%20donated %20gametes,for%20single%20men%20or%20women.

Centers for Disease Control (n.d.-a). *Infertility FAQs*. Retrieved September 24, 2022, from https://www.cdc.gov/reproductivehealth/infertility/

Centers for Disease Control (n.d.-b). *Stillbirth*. Retrieved October 14, 2022, from https://www.cdc.gov/ncbddd/stillbirth/facts.html

Choe, J., Archer, J.S., & Shanks, A.L. (2022, May 1). *In vitro fertilization*. National Institute of Health: National Library of Medicine. https://www.ncbi.nlm.nih.gov/books/NBK562266/

Cleveland Clinic (n.d.-a). *Azoospermia*. Retrieved October 16, 2022, from https://my.clevelandclinic.org/health/diseases/15441-azoospermia

Cleveland Clinic (n.d.-b). *Chemical pregnancy*. Retrieved October 16, 2022, from https://my.clevelandclinic.org/health/diseases/22188-chemical-pregnancy

Cleveland Clinic (n.d.-c). *Conception*. Retrieved October 20, 2022, from https://my.clevelandclinic.org/health/articles/11585-conception

Dugas, C., & Slane, V.H. (2022, June 27). *Miscarriage*. National Library of Medicine: National Institutes of Health. https://www.ncbi.nlm.nih.gov/books/NBK532992/

Helo, S. (2022, May 24). *Abnormal sperm morphology: What does it mean?* Mayo Clinic. https://www.mayoclinic.org/diseases-conditions/male-infertility/expert-answers/sperm-morphology/faq-20057760#:~:text=Normal%20sperm%20have %20an%20oval,misshapen%20sperm%20isn%27t%20uncommon

Johns Hopkins Medicine (n.d.). *Infertility risk factors for men and women*. Retrieved September 24, 2022, from https://www.hopkinsmedicine.org/health/conditions-and-diseases/infertility-risk-factors-for-men-and-women

Johnson, S. (2017, July 2). *Semen analysis and test results*. Healthline. https://www.healthline.com/health/semen-analysis

Kaiser Permanente (2020, February 11). *Gamete and zygote intrafallopian transfer (GIFT and ZIFT) for infertility*. https://wa.kaiserpermanente.org/kbase/topic.jhtml?docId=hw202763

Lee J.K., & Khan, C. (2021). Abortion. In Chou, B., Bienstock, J.L., & Satin, A.J. (Eds.). *The Johns Hopkins manual of gynecology and obstetrics* (6th ed., pp. 386–390). Wolters Kluwer Health.

March of Dimes (n.d.-a). *Birth defects and your baby*. Retrieved September 24, 2022, from https://www.marchofdimes.org/complications/birth-defects-and-your-baby.aspx

March of Dimes (n.d.-b). *Neonatal death*. Retrieved September 24, 2022, from https://www.marchofdimes.org/complications/neonatal-death.aspx

Mayo Clinic (2021a, April 14). *Premature birth*. https://www.mayoclinic.org/diseases-conditions/premature-birth/symptoms-causes/syc-20376730

Mayo Clinic (2021b, October 16). *Miscarriage*. https://www.mayoclinic.org/diseases-conditions/pregnancy-loss-miscarriage/symptoms-causes/syc-20354298

Mitchell, C. N. C. & Christianson, M.S. (2021). Infertility and assisted reproductive technologies. In Chou, B., Bienstock, J.L., & Satin, A.J. (Eds.). *The Johns Hopkins manual of gynecology and obstetrics* (6th ed., pp. 507–525). Wolters Kluwer Health.

National Cancer Institute (n.d.-a). *Fertility issues in girls and women with cancer*. National Institutes of Health. Retrieved September 24, 2022, from https://www.cancer.gov/about-cancer/treatment/side-effects/fertility-women#:~:text=Fertility%20Issues%20in%20Girls%20and,girl's%20or%20a%20woman's%20fertility.&text=Many%20cancer%20treatments%20can%20affect,of%2C%20or%20cause%2C%20infertility

National Cancer Institute (n.d.-b). *Transvaginal ultrasound*. National Institutes of Health. Retrieved September 24, 2022, from https://www.cancer.gov/publications/dictionaries/cancer-terms/def/transvaginal-ultrasound

National Institute of Child Health and Human Development (n.d.). *How common is male factor infertility, and what are its causes?* U.S. Department of Health and Human Services: National Institutes of Health. Retrieved September 24, 2022, from https://www.nichd.nih.gov/health/topics/menshealth/conditioninfo/infertility#:~:text=Ovrall%2C%20one%2Dthird%20of%20infertility,issues%20or%20by%20unknown%20facors.&text=To%20conceive%20a%20child%2C%20a,combine%20with%20a%20womans%20egg

NYU Langone Health (n.d.-a). *Surgery for conditions related to female infertility*. Retrieved September 24, 2022, from https://nyulangone.org/conditions/infertility-in-women/treatments/surgery-for-conditions-related-to-infertility-in-women

NYU Langone Health (n.d.-b). *Surgery for male infertility*. Retrieved September 24, 2022, from https://nyulangone.org/conditions/male-infertility/treatments/surgery-for-male-infertility

Rebar, R.W. (2020, September). *Problems with cervical mucus*. Merck Manual. https://www.merckmanuals.com/home/women-s-health-issues/infertility/problems-with-cervical-mucus#:~:text=If%20cervical%20mucus%20is%20abnormal,promote%20the%20destruction%20of%20sperm

Shah, A.A. (2020, September 18). *Frequently asked questions about frozen embryo transfers*. Shady Grove Fertility. https://www.shadygrovefertility.com/article/frequently-asked-questions-about-frozen-embryo-transfers/

Society for Assisted Reproductive Technology (n.d.). *Assisted reproductive technologies*. Retrieved October 12, 2022, from https://www.sart.org/patients/a-patients-guide-to-assisted-reproductive-technology/general-information/assisted-reproductive-technologies/#:~:text=Assisted%20Reproductive%20Technology%20(ART)%20includes,oocyte%20donation%20and%20gestational%20carriers.

The American College of Obstetricians and Gynecologists (2016, May). *Repeated miscarriages*. https://www.acog.org/womens-health/faqs/repeated-miscarriages

The American College of Obstetricians and Gynecologists (2018, February). *Ectopic pregnancy*. https://www.acog.org/womens-health/faqs/ectopic-pregnancy

The American College of Obstetricians and Gynecologists (2019, May 23). *Infertility workup for the women's health specialist*. https://www.acog.org/clinical/clinical-guidance/committee-opinion/articles/2019/06/infertility-workup-for-the-womens-health-specialist

The American College of Obstetricians and Gynecologists (2022, June). *Sterilization for women and men*. https://www.acog.org/womens-health/faqs/sterilization-for-women-and-men

UNC Fertility (n.d.). *Donors and surrogacy: Choosing your path to parenthood*. Retrieved September 24, 2022, from https://uncfertility.com/understanding-fertility/donors-and-surrogacy/

World Health Organization (2020, September 14). *Infertility*. https://www.who.int/news-room/fact-sheets/detail/infertility

Yale Medicine (n.d.). *Ovulation induction and intrauterine insemination*. Retrieved September 24, 2022, from https://www.yalemedicine.org/conditions/ovulation-induction-intrauterine-insemination#:~:text=Ovulation%20induction%20uses%20fertility%20medications,ovulation%20induction%20to%20achieve%20pregnancy.

CHAPTER THREE

Psychological Impacts of Infertility

A Mind That Questions and a Heart That Hurts

In Chapter 2, we explored the biological components of infertility and reproductive loss. We discussed ways in which testing, diagnosis, treatment, and the experience of reproductive loss served as the crisis that sets the hero on her journey. We also pointed out that the biological crisis is a catalyst for other types of challenges. In Chapter 3, we explore how our hero is further separated from her ordinary world and propelled into another type of crisis: a psychological one. A mind that questions and a heart that hurts are the essence of this chapter as we address the deep psychological impact of infertility.

Many people envision having children as part of their transition into adulthood. Desires for parenthood are motivated by various reasons. These include the longing for emotional bonds with children, gratification received from the parent-child relationship, having help in the family and support in old age, expectations from others, and the status that children can provide (Nauck, 2007). Many dream about and plan for the day they will have families of their own. When these dreams do not become reality, both individuals and couples can experience a variety of complex emotions including anxiety, worry, loneliness, guilt, fear, depression, grief, and regret (Hasanpoor-Azghdy et al., 2014). The psychological stress of dealing with infertility has even been likened to that of people coping with other illnesses such as HIV, cancer, heart disease, and chronic pain (Domar et al., 1993). Other problems include reduced self-esteem, feelings of failure, loss of control, hopelessness (Hasanpoor-Azghdy et al., 2014), loss of identity, feelings of defectiveness and incompetence, anger, marital problems, feelings of worthlessness (Deka & Sarma, 2010), and sexual dysfunction (Starc et al., 2019). And because of the traumatic nature of recurrent loss associated with infertility, many women even develop posttraumatic stress disorder (Roozitalab et al., 2022).

DOI: 10.4324/9781003336402-5

While infertility in itself can cause much psychological strain, social expectations related to parenthood, tension in the partner relationship due to infertility, financial burdens resulting from the cost of treatment, and even the infertility treatments themselves can amplify impacts on emotional health and wellbeing. Compounding these challenges, the variety of emotions experienced may also negatively impact individuals and their relationships. We'll delve more into the social, or relational, crisis in Chapter 4, but for now, we explore three aspects of the psychological crisis. These include crises of grief, psychological disorders, and complex emotions.

THE CRISIS OF GRIEF

Grief, a reaction commonly associated with death, is also a common response for those experiencing infertility. Many different types of grief exist. We'll explore those later in this chapter, but first, let's examine the differences between grief, mourning, and bereavement.

Grief

Grief is a natural reaction to loss characterized by strong and sometimes overwhelming feelings of sadness, numbness, and being removed from daily life (Mayo Clinic, 2016). While some definitions describe grief as a reaction to someone's death, the loss can come in many forms including the loss of a job, the loss of a relationship, or the loss of a dream. When it comes to infertility and reproductive loss, grief often begins with the loss of dreams associated with parenthood. But this is just one of many losses that occur.

As helping professionals, the traditional understanding of grief for a couple who has experienced miscarriage or stillbirth may be more immediately recognizable. We are more likely to empathize and even sympathize with the grief associated with death. However, it is imperative for you to remember that those who are unable to conceive grieve no less than those who have become pregnant and then lost their babies. They grieve what might have been. They grieve what will never be. And when you hear someone say, "They were never able to have children," you can rest assured it was never as simple as that.

Some may wonder how those suffering from infertility can experience such ongoing grief when they never really had anything to lose in the first place. Ah, touché. There are oh, so many losses to grieve. Here are just a few examples. They grieve the loss of their identity (Who am I if I'm not a mother?). They grieve the loss of the way they thought their lives would turn out (married with children and a white picket fence). They grieve the loss of dreams they had (visits from Santa and the Easter Bunny). They grieve the loss of expected milestones (positive pregnancy tests, gender reveals, baby showers, giving birth, first steps, first words, and the first day of school). They grieve the loss of this wonderful, exciting, challenging, hardest-job-you'll-ever-love thing called parenthood. And, by default, that means losing grandparenthood, too.

This is just the beginning. Other types of grief may come into play. What if a person's family doesn't recognize the loss? What if they don't support the person in the grieving process? What if the grief doesn't get any better and turns into a chronic problem? One thing we repeat in this book is that every story is different. While we attempt to describe various reactions to loss, please keep in mind that grief and sorrow manifest themselves in many ways. We encourage you to tune in to each individual story and the way grief is experienced and displayed in each unique situation.

Mourning

Mourning is the act of sorrowing (Merriam-Webster, n.d.-c). It is an expression of deep sadness shown by someone who is grieving. This is often characterized by outward displays of sorrow and is action-oriented. Examples include talking about the loss, crying, or wearing black clothing. While these expressions may be common for those who have experienced death, when it comes to infertility, you won't see many people outwardly mourning their losses. This very private and personal struggle is not usually discussed openly, and therefore, grief is not expressed openly. Mourning may be more common in cases of miscarriage and stillbirth, especially if sources of social support were aware of the pregnancy.

Bereavement

Bereavement is a state or condition of having experienced a loss or being deprived of someone or something (Merriam-Webster, n.d.-a). Bereavement is often associated with a specific time period, usually when sadness and pain are at their highest levels. This period varies greatly from person to person. There is no timetable for how long it will last. Some people start to feel better in a few weeks. For some, it takes months and even years. For those experiencing infertility and reproductive loss, it can be much longer, perhaps indefinitely, especially if losses are ongoing. While grief, mourning, and bereavement are closely related, for the purposes of this book, we focus on grief. Now let's explore the five basic reactions to loss and examine seven different types of grief.

Five Basic Reactions to Loss

No matter what the person's story is, you, in your role as the helping professional, may find some common threads woven throughout grieving experiences. Elizabeth Kubler-Ross, in her seminal work on death and dying, developed a model describing what happens when people grieve (Kubler-Ross, 1969). Since the development of this framework, other models have emerged. These include Bowlby and Parkes's Four Phases of Grief, Worden's Four Basic Tasks in Adapting to Loss, Wolfelt's Companioning Approach to Grieving, and Neimeyer's Narrative and Constructivist Model (Tyrrell et al., 2022). We refer to these works to broaden your understanding of grief. However, for the purpose of this book, we're using Kubler-Ross's well-known landmark model to frame the discussion because our emphasis is on the psychological crisis, not how the person moves through grief. Kubler-Ross's model includes five stages: denial, anger, bargaining, depression, and acceptance. Those struggling with infertility and reproductive loss can move in and out of these stages in no particular order, and even if someone reaches the acceptance stage, life happens, memories or emotions get triggered, and the person may revert to some of the previous stages. Let's look at a few examples of the thoughts and feelings associated with each stage.

Stage 1 is the denial stage. It involves a state of disbelief surrounding the loss. For those experiencing infertility, denial may manifest itself in statements such as, "This can't be happening to me. I've always been so healthy!" or that unfailing hope that next month everything will work out, not recognizing a deeper problem.

Stage 2 is the anger stage. This anger could be directed at any number of targets including oneself, others, or God. In this stage, someone may have a thought like, "It's not fair! How can people who abuse their children get pregnant so easily, but people like me, who can provide a loving home, can't?"

Stage 3 is the bargaining stage. Bargaining usually consists of statements related to what the person wishes they had or had not done such as, "I wish I had started trying for kids at a much younger age" or vowing to get healthy, eat organically, and start exercising regularly.

Stage 4 is the depression stage. It involves acute sadness that may begin to interfere with everyday life. Someone who is depressed about the inability to conceive may say, "This is hopeless. My life won't be worth living if I never have children."

Finally, Stage 5 is the acceptance stage. At this stage, people accept the reality of their losses. Someone suffering from infertility who has reached the acceptance stage may say, "It just wasn't meant to be. Maybe I can find a new purpose for my life and move on." See Figure 3.1 for a diagram of Kubler-Ross's grief cycle.

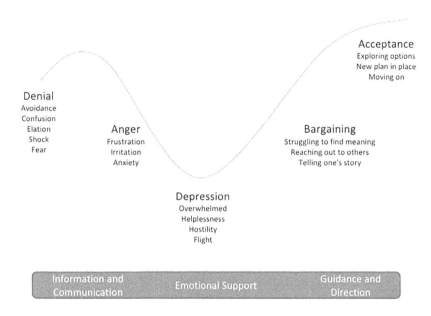

FIGURE 3.1 The Kübler-Ross Grief Cycle

Source: https://commons.wikimedia.org/wiki/File:Kubler-ross-grief-cycle-1-728.jpg#filelinks

Some will move through Kubler-Ross's grief stages as outlined, however, many do not. Some may experience other types of grief including complex reactions that hinder the healing process. These include abbreviated grief, ambiguous grief, complicated grief, chronic sorrow, disenfranchised grief, secondary losses, and traumatic grief. Let's review those now.

Abbreviated Grief

Abbreviated grief is a type of grief that passes relatively quickly or more quickly than expected (Epstein, 2021). This type of grief may occur for several reasons. First, the grief may be short-lived because the loss was imminent, and the person grieved in anticipation. Grieving in anticipation is referred to as anticipatory grief (Eldridge, 2021). For example, a woman who had a ruptured appendix in childhood may have known for many years that natural conception was unlikely. When a reproductive endocrinologist confirms this to be true, she grieves for a short time but then quickly moves into exploring alternative options for parenthood. Second, abbreviated grief may occur because there wasn't a sense of attachment to what was lost. For example, a man's grief related to his wife's ectopic pregnancy was brief because he hadn't yet developed an emotional connection with the child. Finally, grief may be abbreviated when something new quickly replaces the thing that was lost. For example, a woman might grieve when the results of her pregnancy test are negative. However, in a few days, she realizes the results were wrong when she retakes the test and gets a positive result.

Ambiguous Grief

Ambiguous grief occurs when there is a lack of information or closure surrounding the loss (Ryder, 2022). This loss may be commonly experienced in individuals who experience unexplained infertility. Maybe doctors performed test after test and can still find no physical problems or issues that would prevent conception. Perhaps someone gives birth to a stillborn child with no explanation for why. The reasons remain unresolved, closure is difficult to achieve, and grief becomes more complex.

Complicated Grief

Complicated grief occurs when a response to loss differs significantly from normal expectations and includes three types: absent grief, delayed grief, and chronic grief (American Psychological Association, n.d.). First, people sometimes don't experience any type of grief. This is called absent grief because the person shows few or no signs. Some believe this is related to the shock or denial associated with the loss as mentioned previously in the discussion of Kubler-Ross's model.

Second, delayed grief occurs much later than expected, maybe even months and years after the loss (Rowe, 2022). This type of grief tends to manifest itself when people suppress their pain. Social and/or professional obligations following the loss and busyness related to taking care of responsibilities such as funeral arrangements may distract the person from experiencing emotions that are typical. The grief tends to emerge later when the person slows down and has time and space to process the loss. Sudden reminders of the loss can also trigger a delayed grief reaction (Rowe, 2022).

Finally, chronic grief is characterized by prolonged or extremely intense grief (American Psychological Association, n.d.). In some cases, losses are especially devastating, and the passage of time doesn't alleviate painful emotions or restore adequate functioning. This is the most common type of complicated grief.

Chronic Sorrow

Continual losses can compound and complicate the grieving process. When this occurs, it is sometimes referred to as chronic sorrow, which is a reaction to loss that isn't final and continues to be present in the life of the griever (Lindgren et al., 1992). When the pain is still present, it's hard to move forward. And even when the person tries to move forward, memories of the loss are still prevalent. The hurt never fully goes away. Features of chronic sorrow include both external and internal stimuli that trigger feelings of loss and disappointment, cyclic sadness that extends over time in a situation that seems to have no end, and intensification of the sadness years after the initial loss (Lindgren et al., 1992). For the hero, constant reminders such as a pregnancy announcement posted on social media or an invitation to a baby shower may trigger feelings of pain and loss. These triggers can stir up negative thoughts and emotions and further complicate the grieving process.

Disenfranchised Grief

Disenfranchised grief is a type of grief that occurs when the loss is not societally recognized or acknowledged (Doka, 1989, 1999, 2002). For example, when a loved one dies, the funeral is a custom that helps bring closure. People send flowers and cards. They visit the home and take food to the family. When it comes to infertility, there are no such rituals or customs to acknowledge the loss or the griever's pain. This can make the griever feel like the loss was invalid or insignificant. Sometimes a person's friends or closest family members don't even offer condolences or words of encouragement. This is a type of secondary loss that can also bring about feelings of isolation which complicate grief.

KEISHA'S STORY

Never once in my life did I ever dream I'd have trouble getting pregnant. My husband and I tried for nine months before our daughter came along. But at the age of 34, I knew I didn't have a whole lot of time left on the fertility clock. We started trying immediately after the doctor cleared us to, and months went by. Then years. For five years, we tried every type of fertility treatment available except in vitro fertilization. It was just too expensive, and we didn't feel right about taking out a loan on something that was a gamble at best. So, at the age of 40, we threw in the towel and stopped trying. It was at this point I really started to grieve. The five years of infertility treatments were filled with hope that it might still happen. But when I stopped treatment, I lost all hope because I pretty much knew it wouldn't. That's when it got bad, especially when several people in my close circle of friends and family got pregnant. At that point, I spiraled into a deep depression because I knew I was going to have to be around all the baby bumps and baby showers and baby cries ... for years and years to come. These were constant reminders of my infertility and the hurt and pain I felt for so long. While I could avoid many situations involving babies, I couldn't avoid these people. It all hit too close to home. Their happiness magnified my sadness; their joy magnified my pain. And many times I would curl up in the fetal position and cry in my bed for hours at a time. I was useless to my husband and daughter when this happened.

It feels like a unique situation because my struggle was with secondary infertility. When you have just one child, other people assume that's all you wanted. They don't know it can hurt just as much as if you never had any. And while I feel bad even saying this, sometimes I think it may hurt worse. Don't get me wrong. I know it must be so painful to long for and never have any children of your own. But this is a different kind of hurt because I grieve a different kind of loss - not of what I'll never have - but of what I'll never have again. I know the joy of carrying a baby and feeling it move and holding it in my arms for the first time. So I grieve that I'll never feel those things again. First words and first steps are the last first words and steps my husband and I will ever experience. The first day of kindergarten was the last first day of kindergarten we'll ever celebrate. So even in the midst of happy moments, an undertone of sadness lingers. I also grieve that my daughter will never have siblings. I grieve that we'll never have big family dinners and holiday gatherings. I grieve that my husband and daughter have to live with me in the midst of my grief. My daughter sometimes asks why I cry all the time. My husband, while supportive, says he misses the glow I used to have. I love my daughter so much, and she brings me so much joy, yet I still feel so sad because I'll never have another.

It doesn't help that nobody ever says anything to me about this. I can't tell you how often I've cried at family gatherings because of all the babies that were there. How many times do you think anybody asked me how I was? How many times did they embrace me to comfort me? How many times did they acknowledge that it must be hard? None. In all the years I've been dealing with this, only one or two people have ever said they were sorry. I know it's awkward for them. I know they don't want to make me feel worse. What they don't realize is that saying nothing makes it worse because it feels like they don't care.

Secondary Losses

Secondary loss occurs when a primary loss triggers subsequent losses. Whether the person realizes it or not, these secondary losses contribute to the pain stemming from the original loss. Secondary losses can manifest themselves in many ways. For example, Jasmine attempts to adopt her foster child, but the adoption fails because the child is suddenly returned to her birth family. Jasmine may grieve the loss of the dreams she had for this child. She may experience a loss of faith because God did not answer her prayers for the adoption to go through. Perhaps her family doesn't acknowledge her grief and tells her to just get over it, which feels like a loss of her support system. Secondary losses can be overwhelming and difficult to navigate in the midst of an already challenging situation. It is important to be aware of and acknowledge grief resulting from all the subsequent losses that stem from the initial loss.

Traumatic Grief

Finally, traumatic grief occurs when a person perceives a loss as horrifying, unexpected, violent, and/or traumatic (Phillips, 2021). Traumatic grief can be associated with both infertility and reproductive loss. When it comes to infertility, perhaps the horrifying experience is getting negative results on pregnancy tests month after month, year after year. When it comes to reproductive loss, the unexpected event may be a miscarriage following a car accident or a fall. The situation could become even more violent and horrifying if the person witnesses large amounts of blood and tissue expelled from the body. Finally, perhaps a mother has no indication that her baby will be stillborn. Pregnancy and labor progressed normally until the actual birth. Then, suddenly, she holds a lifeless child in her arms. Each of these experiences can be traumatizing and may lead to memories that are especially problematic. These individuals may need special consideration and perhaps even screenings for and treatment of posttraumatic stress disorder.

While grief related to infertility and reproductive loss is heartbreaking, many sufferers do end up having children. Some conceive, some adopt, and some choose surrogacy. However, just because the quest seems over, the emotional wounds and scars do not go away. Many people feel the ripple effects of hurt and pain long after they become parents. Sometimes, those struggling with infertility never have children. No matter how the story ends, grief is only one aspect of the psychological crisis. Another is the crisis of psychological disorders.

THE CRISIS OF PSYCHOLOGICAL DISORDERS

Sometimes, grief-related infertility leads to deeper psychological problems. These include the development of psychological disorders. Commonly diagnosed disorders related to infertility and reproductive loss include anxiety, depression, post-traumatic stress disorder, and prolonged grief disorder.

Anxiety

Anxiety is a common emotion experienced by those struggling with infertility, with the results of one study indicating that 86% of infertile women suffered (Ramezanzadeh et al., 2004). According to the Diagnostic and Statistical Manual of Mental Disorders (American Psychiatric Association, 2022), the disorder is characterized by excessive worry that is difficult to control and is associated with restlessness, fatigue, difficulty concentrating, irritability, muscle tension, and/or sleep disturbance. While anxiety, which is associated with uncertainty about the future, is a normal part of life for most people, it can intensify based on the situation. When it comes to infertility and reproductive loss, the outcome is always uncertain. Will this pregnancy test be positive? Will I get pregnant this month? Will I get pregnant this year? Will I ever get pregnant? Will these medications make me feel crazy? Will this procedure be painful? Will I miscarry again? Will this baby be born alive? Will I ever have a child of my own? The questions are numerous. And endless. And the answers are few. Not knowing the outcome, as well as the feeling of powerlessness to change the situation can be extremely difficult, especially when someone wants something so badly. In severe cases, the worry may interfere with everyday life. Sufferers may not be able to concentrate on anything but fertility and fertility treatments. These emotions may persist for long periods of time and can even induce feelings of panic.

Depression

Depression is also commonly experienced by those suffering from infertility. Results of one study indicated that 40.8% of infertile women were depressed (Ramezanzadeh et al., 2004). Depression is characterized by depressed mood, diminished interest or pleasure in activities, weight loss or gain, a slowing down of thought or movement, fatigue, feelings of worthlessness or guilt, inability to concentrate, and even recurrent thoughts of death (American Psychiatric Association, 2022). Depression is often exacerbated by other issues. The stress, shame, secrecy, and ongoing disappointment and frustration of infertility can worsen the condition. Feelings of sadness, grief, and sorrow can complicate the disorder. The diagnosis of other medical conditions can also contribute.

Infertility treatments themselves may induce or exacerbate depression. Medications used to treat infertility often involve the use of hormones which can disrupt bodily processes, cause mood swings, and contribute to depressive symptoms. The emotional and physical challenges of repetitive, costly, invasive treatments can increase both depression and anxiety. This emotional strain can negatively impact relationships and compound depressive symptoms. Lack of social support can worsen the problem or prevent improvement.

Posttraumatic Stress Disorder

In some cases, women who experience infertility and reproductive loss develop posttraumatic stress disorder. Results of one study indicated that 41.3% of infertile women had symptoms (Roozitalab et al., 2022). The disorder is characterized by exposure to trauma that leads to intrusive thoughts and reactions such as upsetting memories, nightmares, or flashbacks. It is also characterized by avoidance of trauma-related stimuli, negative thoughts or feelings that began or worsened following the trauma, and arousal and reactivity that began or worsened after the trauma including irritability or aggression, destructive behavior, hypervigilance, and difficulty concentrating or sleeping (American Psychiatric Association, 2022). The fear, helplessness, and horror of infertility and reproductive loss, often experienced over a number of years, provide more than enough trauma to lead to the development of this disorder. And triggers such as a diaper commercial on television or a crying baby in a grocery store can send the sufferer into an emotional tailspin, even years later.

Prolonged Grief Disorder

Earlier in this chapter, we discussed various types of grief reactions. In some cases, a person's grief lasts beyond what is socially, culturally, or religiously expected. Prolonged grief disorder is a disorder that is diagnosed when at least one year has passed since a loss has occurred, and the loss begins to interfere with daily functioning (American Psychiatric Association, 2022). Symptoms include loss of identity, a sense of disbelief, intense emotional pain, avoidance of things that are reminders of the loss, loneliness, and feelings that life is meaningless. The challenges of infertility can be exacerbated by the roller coaster ride of hope and loss experienced by individuals month after month, year after year. Consider the person who has 53 negative pregnancy tests or seven miscarriages. From their perspective, it may seem that grief will never end.

As we end this section on the crisis of psychological disorders, we'd like to point out that some individuals may develop anxiety, depression, post-traumatic stress disorder, and prolonged grief disorder because of the infertility experience. However, many may suffer from mental health issues prior to beginning the journey. For those who already deal with these challenges, symptoms can intensify. For those who struggle with other diagnoses such as bipolar disorder or eating disorders, the experience of infertility may have a compounding effect. You, the helping professional, must remain mindful of how these challenges can impact your hero's journey. But even if psychological disorders never come into play, your hero will certainly encounter another type of crisis, the crisis of complex emotions.

THE CRISIS OF COMPLEX EMOTIONS

While people suffering from infertility may develop psychological disorders, they may also experience a wide variety of complex and challenging emotions. These include loss of identity, feelings of defectiveness, incompetence, worthlessness, anger, marital problems (Deka & Sarma, 2010), and social isolation (Gokler et al., 2014).

Loss of Identity and Feelings of Defectiveness, Incompetence, and Worthlessness

Those struggling with infertility may experience a loss of identity as well as feelings of defectiveness, incompetence, and worthlessness. First, let's explore the loss of identity. Identity is the distinguished personality or character of an individual (Merriam-Webster, n.d.-b). For some, identity is found in money, popularity, grades, or athletic ability. For those suffering from infertility, identity is often related to parenthood, so when the parenting role is not achieved, a crisis can occur. Perhaps a woman married young and chose not to attend college because she planned on becoming a stay-at-home mom. When she's unable to conceive, she wonders what her purpose in life really is and begins to doubt that she can do anything else. Identity is sometimes related to feelings of defectiveness, incompetence, and worthlessness. Notions such as these may invade when someone's body won't function the way they thought it should or when conception is so difficult but seems so easy for others. Thoughts such as these can intensify already complex emotions and contribute to decreased self-esteem and feelings of inferiority.

Anger

We already mentioned anger in the section on Kubler-Ross's five reactions to loss, but we felt the need to address it again here. Anger can come in many forms, including anger at self and others. Examples include anger toward one's own body, anger with God, or anger with other women who seem to conceive easily. Anger may also be closely associated with feelings of guilt and self-blame.

Consider the following scenarios. Sharon feels both guilty and angry with herself for contracting a sexually transmitted infection that led to her infertility. Jade blames herself for being unable to carry on the family name. Matteo feels guilty about not being able to give a child to his partner who desperately wants children. Russell blames himself for not trying to start a family sooner and gets angry with those who told him he should wait to have children. These thoughts and experiences are common. Other feelings such as doubt and shame may also prevail. "Maybe I'm not cut out to be a parent." "My body is broken and defective". "What if my partner stops loving me if I can't give him a child?" These types of recurring thoughts and emotions can take their toll on mental well-being.

Marital Problems

Infertility can also have a negative impact on the couple's relationship (Deka & Sarma, 2010). Problems with a spouse or partner can add to an already volatile emotional situation caused by infertility. Partners may feel anxious about conception which can increase sexual dysfunction and isolation. They may disagree about medical decisions, how much money to spend on treatment, and how much or how little to tell others about their infertility. Discord in the relationship can further contribute to feelings of anger, self-blame, and doubt. You'll learn more about the negative impact on the partner relationship in Chapter 4 where we examine the social crisis of infertility.

Social Isolation

Finally, social isolation is common for those suffering from infertility. Social support from close relationships is a vital resource for coping with stress (Hostinar & Gunnar, 2015). Because infertility can be an extremely stressful situation, those who suffer would benefit from a strong support system. However, infertility can sometimes cause the sufferer to feel very alone. It is a very personal, private issue involving intimate details of a person's life. After all, when someone asks how you are, do you really want to say, "Great! I drove to the doctor's office this morning with a cup of semen between my legs!"? In addition, there is a certain amount of stigma associated with not being able to have children. Avoiding social situations, especially involving those with babies, is not uncommon. And friends and family members often do not know how to offer aid. Sometimes they even leave the sufferer out of special events and gatherings for fear of making them uncomfortable or upset. Therefore, people struggling with infertility may lack the social support they need to both comfort and guide them through the crisis. They often feel alone. This isolation adds to the already stressful experience of infertility.

CONCLUSION

Well, we're two for three. In Chapter 2, we learned about the biological crisis of infertility. In this chapter, we explored the psychological crisis including the crisis of grief, the crisis of psychological disorders, and the crisis of complex emotions. We hope you now have a better understanding of some of the mental and emotional struggles of those experiencing infertility and reproductive loss. Since we've already discussed the biological and psychological crises of infertility, in Chapter 4, we end with the third piece of the puzzle, the social crisis.

REFERENCES

American Psychiatric Association. (2022). *Diagnostic and statistical manual of mental disorders* (5th ed., text revision). American Psychiatric Association Publishing.

American Psychological Association (n.d.). *APA dictionary of psychology: Complicated grief*. Retrieved September 25, 2022, from https://dictionary.apa.org/complicated-grief

Deka, P.K. & Sarma, S. (2010). Psychological aspects of infertility. *British Journal of Medical Practitioners*, *3*(3), a336.

Doka, K.J. (1989). *Disenfranchised grief: Recognizing hidden sorrow*. Lexington, MA: Lexington Books.

Doka, K.J. (1999). Disenfranchised grief. *Bereavement Care*, *18*, 37–39. doi: 10.1080/02682629908657467

Doka, K.J. (2002). *Disenfranchised grief: New challenges, directions, and strategies for practice*. Champaign, IL: Research Press.

Domar A.D., Zuttermeister, P.C., and Friedman, R. (1993). The psychological impact of infertility: A comparison with patients with other medical conditions. *Journal of Psychosomatic Obstetrics and Gynecology, 14*, 45–52.

Eldridge, L. (2021). *How anticipatory grief differs from grief after death*. VeryWellHealth. https://www.verywellhealth.com/understanding-anticipatory-grief-and-symptoms-2248855

Epstein, S. (2021). *Three reasons we may not grieve a big loss: How to understand and accept abbreviated grief*. Psychology Today. https://www.psychologytoday.com/us/blog/between-the-generations/202103/3-reasons-we-might-not-grieve-big-loss

Gokler, M.E., Unsal, A., & Arslantis, D. (2014). The prevalence of infertility and loneliness among women aged 18–49 years who are living in semi-rural areas in western Turkey. *International Journal of Fertility and Sterility, 8*(2), 155–162.

Hasanpoor-Azghdy, S.B., Simbar, M., & Vedadhir, A. (2014). The emotional-psychological consequences among infertile women seeking treatment: The results of a qualitative study. *Iranian Journal of Reproductive Medicine*, *12*(2), 131–138.

Hostinar, C. E. & Gunnar, M.R. (2015). Social support can buffer against stress and shape brain activity. *AJOB Neuroscience*, *6*(3), 34–42. 10.1080/21507740. 2015.1047054

Kubler-Ross, E. (1969). *On death and dying*. Scribner.

Lindgren, C.L., Burke, M.L., Hainsworth, M.A., & Eakes, G.G. (1992). Chronic sorrow: A lifespan concept. *Scholarly Inquiry for Nursing Practice*, *6*(1), 27–40.

Mayo Clinic (2016). *What is grief?* https://www.mayoclinic.org/patient-visitor-guide/support-groups/what-is-grief

Merriam-Webster (n.d.-a). *Bereavement*. Retrieved September 25, 2022, from https://www.merriam-webster.com/dictionary/bereavement

Merriam-Webster (n.d.-b). *Identity*. Retrieved October 8, 2022, from https://www.merriam-webster.com/dictionary/identity

Merriam-Webster (n.d.-c). *Mourning*. Retrieved September 25, 2022, from https://www.merriam-webster.com/dictionary/mourning

Nauck, B. (2007). Value of children and the framing of fertility: Results from a cross-cultural comparative survey in 10 societies. *European Sociological Review*, *23*(5), 615–629.

Phillips, L. (2021, May 4). *Untangling trauma and grief after loss*. Counseling Today. https://ct.counseling.org/2021/05/untangling-trauma-and-grief-after-loss/

Ramezanzadeh, F., Aghssa, M.M., Abedinia, N., Zayeri, F., Khanafshar, N., Shariat, M., & Jafarabadi, M. (2004). A survey of relationship between anxiety, depression, and duration of infertility. *BMC Women's Health*, *4*(9). 10.1186/1472-6874-4-9

Roozitalab, S., Rahimzadeh, M., Mirmajidi, S.R., Ataee, M., & Saeieh, S.E. (2022). The relationship between infertility, stress, and quality of life with posttraumatic stress disorder in infertile women. *Journal of Reproductive Infertility*, *22*(4), 282–288. 10.18502/jri.v22i4.7654

Rowe, S. (2022). *Delayed grief: Causes, symptoms, and how to cope*. PsychCentral. https://psychcentral.com/health/delayed-grief

Ryder, G. (2022). *Ambiguous grief: Mourning without closure*. PsychCentral. https://psychcentral.com/health/ambiguous-grief

Starc, A., Trampuš, M., Jukić, D.P., Grgas-Bile, C., Jukić, T., & Mivšek, A.P. (2019). Infertility and sexual dysfunctions: A systematic literature review. *Acta Clinica Croatia*, *58*(3), 508–515. 10.20471/acc.2019.58.03.15

Tyrrell, P., Harberger, S., Schoo, C., & Siddiqui, W. (2022). *Kubler-Ross stages of dying and subsequent models of grief*. National Library of Medicine: National Institutes of Health. https://www.ncbi.nlm.nih.gov/books/NBK507885/

CHAPTER FOUR

Social Impacts of Infertility

One Is the Loneliest Number

In Chapter 3, we explored psychological struggles related to infertility. Closely intertwined with the psychological impact is the social impact related to the condition. In the previous chapter, we touched on the relevance of social support in the hero's process. We explored how positive social support aids in combating stress, and the lack of this support can contribute to a sense of isolation. Throughout Chapter 4, we further explore how the hero's relationships are affected by their struggle with infertility and reproductive loss.

No matter what path we travel in life, we all need mentors who can provide support and encouragement during challenging events and circumstances. For those suffering from infertility, physicians and specialists are often viewed as a first-line source of information and support. Yet many sufferers report a lack of empathy and compassion from them along with a lack of clarity regarding potential outcomes.

Unfortunately, because infertility is such a private journey, typical sources of social support are often unaware of the person's plight, and, therefore, do not offer aid. Even if sufferers do discuss their struggles openly, they may be met with limited understanding. These often well-intentioned individuals don't know how it feels. They don't know what to say. They don't know what to do. And ultimately, they may even do more harm than good, especially if they say nothing, offer hollow platitudes, or even turn their backs on those who confide in them. These reactions may prevent the sufferer from confiding in others in the future. The social crisis of infertility can negatively impact relationships. Let's explore this further by looking at the way it can impact relationships with spouses and partners, friends and family, faith, and even self.

DOI: 10.4324/9781003336402-6

RELATIONSHIPS WITH A SPOUSE OR PARTNER

Social support is the best buffer to cushion people against the impact of stress in their lives (Hostinar & Gunnar, 2015). Some are fortunate to have the support of a spouse or partner to stand by them throughout the roller coaster ride of the ordeal. Some people even believe that the experience of infertility brought them closer to their partner because of the shared experience. However, infertility can also lead to problems in a marriage or partner relationships. Results of one study indicated that women who don't have children after pursuing infertility treatment are three times more likely to end cohabitation with their partner or to divorce than those who do (Kjaer et al., 2014). Infertility can negatively impact the partner relationship in several ways. These include sexual intimacy, emotional strain, lack of support outside the relationship, feelings of inadequacy, and disagreements.

Sexual Intimacy

Sexual intimacy shared between couples can bring them closer together. Sex can also cause division and stress when viewed in the context of infertility. Results of multiple studies indicated that infertility negatively impacted sexual self-esteem, sexual relationships, and sexual functioning (Tao et al., 2011). Similarly, the stress of infertility seems to directly decrease sexual self-esteem, the frequency of sexual intercourse, and satisfaction with one's own sexual performance (Andrews et al., 1991).

Sexual difficulties can occur for several reasons. Because ovulation takes place only once a month, sex must often be planned. This can take away from spontaneity and intimacy. It may also create pressure to perform. This pressure may inhibit sexual response and induce feelings of anxiety more than pleasure. What if the male partner is unable to obtain an erection or achieve orgasm? The female partner may feel angry and even place blame on her partner because the opportunity for conception that month is so limited. Similarly, what if the day has arrived for an intrauterine insemination procedure? The male must masturbate into a cup, then someone must transport the cup to the specialist's office (usually by holding it between the legs, in the waistband, or in the bra while driving) and drop it off with a receptionist. Sounds intimate, right? And what if the man is unable to provide the sample that day? A lot of time and money have gone into preparing for the procedure only to have no sperm available to make it all happen. Tension and resentment may build.

In addition, a once joyful act with freedom of mind and body may now be accompanied by undertones of anxiety or sadness. Sex could be a trigger, a constant reminder of the pain associated with infertility. Consider the following scenarios. A man says his partner loves him and is fulfilled in their sexual relationship, but he senses her continual sadness and never feels like she can let go and enjoy it because sex is a constant reminder of her inability to conceive. A woman cries after sex wondering why two people who love each other so much are unable to have children. A woman's anxiety increases during sex because intimate touching by her partner reminds her of the uncomfortable procedure she experienced the previous week during her fertility treatment. Or, a couple may enjoy their sex life immensely, but their doctor directs them to limit sex before or after procedures. A joyful act that once united these couples is now filled with hurt, pain, and frustration that divides.

Emotional Strain

Ongoing emotional strain can erode a couple's relationship. Anxiety, depression, and a sense of hopelessness and helplessness can interfere with the happiness and joy that may have once permeated the relationship. The stress of infertility increases marital conflict (Andrews et al., 1991) and leads to greater dissatisfaction in marriage (Javaid et al., 2022). Couples may feel sad. They may cry. They may get angry with the situation or with each other. They may obsess over the baby they so desperately long for. They may worry about how it will all turn out. They may fear never becoming parents. And if they are undergoing treatment for infertility, the stress of treatment itself can be detrimental to the relationship. Doctor appointments, medications and their emotional side effects, tests, and procedures can be time-consuming, expensive, and wreak havoc on the body. When the focus of the relationship is conception, the couple may, unfortunately, neglect other important aspects of their union. And if conception never occurs, childlessness may serve as a constant reminder of their pain.

Other sources of strain include lack of support from a partner, lack of support outside the partner relationship, feelings of inadequacy, and disagreements. Lack of support from a partner can have detrimental impacts. A person struggling with infertility may expect one person in their life - their partner - to relate to the situation more than anyone else. However, some individuals may have partners who don't express care or empathy because they may process the experience differently. They may not understand why it matters so much. Perhaps their desire for children was not as strong. This lack of understanding and empathy can add to a sense of isolation, perhaps even resentment.

Lack of Support Outside the Relationship and Feelings of Inadequacy

Lack of support outside the relationship and feelings of inadequacy can also cause strain. Because couples may not have much external social support, the partner may become an emotional dumping ground. This can be a difficult load to bear and can add more stress to an already tense situation. In addition, tension can increase if one member of the relationship feels a sense of inadequacy related to the situation. For example, a husband may want to fix his wife's sadness and doesn't know how. Perhaps the woman is the source of infertility and worries her partner will stop loving her or leave her if she's unable to give him a child.

Disagreements

Difficulties may also arise when couples disagree about decisions related to infertility. For example, they may have very different viewpoints about seeking medical help. Perhaps one is ready to move forward with any and every treatment option available while the other isn't ready to take that path. Maybe one partner wants to adopt, but the other does not. In same-sex couples, there might be disagreement about which partner will be the biological parent. Finally, disagreements could revolve around the financial burden of treatment. Infertility treatments can be very expensive with one full cycle of in vitro fertilization costing around $20,000.00 (Wu et al., 2014). They may disagree on how much they are willing to spend on a treatment that does not have a likelihood of success. Will they dip into a savings account? Will they borrow money from a bank? Will they ask for help from family members?

Maybe they disagree about whether to tell other people, who to tell, or exactly how much information to share. One partner may want to tell their church and ask for prayer while the other partner wants it to be private. One partner may want to confide in friends, while the other is only okay with disclosure to close family. Partners may also disagree about moving forward. Will they continue with treatment? If so, for how long? Will they take a break for a while or keep trudging through? Should they give up and try adoption or surrogacy? Areas of potential disagreement are endless, and the decisions are all high stakes. For partners, infertility and reproductive loss can impact sexual intimacy, cause emotional strain, contribute to feelings of isolation, and lead to disagreements. But the ramifications extend far beyond partner and marriage relationships. Next, let's look at how the condition impacts relationships with friends and family.

RELATIONSHIPS WITH FRIENDS AND FAMILY

For individuals struggling with infertility, relationships with friends and family can be especially difficult. While these individuals can be well-meaning, they sometimes become a source of pain. In addition, social media, intended to bring friends together, can sometimes cause division.

Friends and Family

Social support is an important part of successfully navigating any stressful life event. In the case of infertility, these social connections may come in the form of friends and family members. However, even the people who care about us most may not know how to handle such a sensitive topic. Some may say very little because they don't know what to say. They may even say nothing at all which can further add to a sense of loneliness and isolation. The lack of acknowledgment can make it seem like they don't care when they may just feel uncomfortable because they don't know how to help. They don't want to say anything that might upset the person. They don't want to cause a scene. So, instead, they talk about anything but what the person is going through. Unfortunately, some friends and family members will intentionally say hurtful things, especially if they are angry or jealous for some reason.

Some truly do care and really do try, but even best efforts may consist of hollow platitudes and advice. Well-meaning friends tell miracle baby stories. Parents constantly ask when they are going to become grandparents and make unhelpful suggestions like standing on your head after sex. Others may give advice such as, "You're so busy focusing on what you don't have. Try focusing on what you do have instead," "You can always try again," and one of our personal favorites … "Just relax. It will happen." Yeah. Doesn't help.

Even strangers may ask, "When are you going to have children?" or in the case of secondary infertility, "When are you having more?" And sometimes it's even children themselves who unintentionally make hurtful comments. The hero experiencing secondary infertility may have a child who asks, "When can I have a brother or sister?" or complain, "I never have anybody to play with." One of us even knows a child who announced to her mother, "I like Emma better than you because she has more children than you. When are you going to have more children like Emma?" While hurtful comments such as these are unintentional, they can still pack a punch, especially on a bad day.

Some who suffer from infertility may avoid social situations to avoid the triggers that induce heartache and pain. Some avoid the people who they know will make the most hurtful comments. Some choose not to attend baby showers, birthday parties, and holiday celebrations where they know expectant mothers, babies, and children will be present. This can be a healthy boundary that protects emotional well-being. However, as much as the client may try to distance herself from potentially painful situations, some circumstances are unavoidable. A colleague at work complains about the weight she's gaining with her third pregnancy. A mother excitedly shares the news about her best friend's son who is expecting his first child. A shopping trip with friends unexpectedly leads to a stop at the baby superstore when one of the ladies remembers she needs to buy a shower gift for her neighbor. Sometimes members of our hero's social support network just don't realize what they're saying. Or doing. Or that those things are painful. As helping professionals, you may consider exploring how to guide your clients, supervisees, and/or students through situations such as these. Do they want to say something? If so, what? Should they be direct? Use humor? Or maybe just walk away? Assist your clients in choosing the path that is best for them in their unique set of circumstances.

While some heroes set boundaries of protection and choose to avoid potentially hurtful situations, sometimes it's the friends and family members who choose to avoid the hero. Results of one study indicate that being excluded or ignored was one of the ways others invalidated women's infertility (McBain & Reeves, 2019). Participants in this study reported feeling excluded from society because they didn't fit in with those who chose to remain child-free, and they didn't fit in with those who had children. In addition, many reported being excluded by friends and family members who didn't invite them to events or who simply stayed away. One participant stated, "'It's one thing for me to say that I can't come, and it's another thing for you to not invite me … Just invite, don't exclude me'" (McBain & Reeves, 2019, p. 159).

Some friends, family, or coworkers make hurtful comments or avoid the one suffering from infertility and reproductive loss, but some may not even acknowledge the person's plight. Remember, disenfranchised grief occurs when a loss is not publicly acknowledged. For those experiencing disenfranchised grief related to infertility, a sense of isolation may be compounded because others may not acknowledge the pain. Because the loss is not seen by others, it feels invisible. This can lead to secondary losses such as the loss of a support network. In addition, in some cases, friends and family may not only ignore the pain but even turn against the sufferer because of it. Consider the following scenarios.

- Alden stopped using social media because he wanted to avoid the numerous gender reveals and birth announcements posted by his friends. This helped his emotional state tremendously. But at the same time, he didn't see any of his mother's posts. Since he didn't see the posts, he didn't "like" them, and he didn't comment on them. His mother got angry and didn't speak to him for a week.
- Gabriella made the decision to go out of town the weekend of her sister's baby shower because she didn't want to break down into an ugly cry in front of all the guests. Her brother-in-law told her she was selfish because if she cared at all, she would be there to support her sister on her special day.
- Treva ran into her cousin and her cousin's newborn baby at the local library. When the cousin asked her if she wanted to hold the baby, she politely declined. However, her father called later to say, "What's wrong with you?

What kind of grown woman doesn't want to hold a baby?" Treva was then asked not to attend Thanksgiving dinner because of the way she acted toward her cousin.

For heroes who face this kind of adversity, it becomes even more essential that helping professionals demonstrate empathy and understanding. They may be the only one who does. It may become necessary to work through negative self-talk related to these situations and assist the hero with finding other sources of social support who can demonstrate care and concern and provide encouragement.

IMANI'S STORY

My whole life changed when I was diagnosed with infertility. At first, it wasn't so bad. I just figured with a little help from my doctor, we'd get this baby thing figured out. After all, I'd never heard anyone else say they'd struggled with getting pregnant. It wasn't even on my radar.

But after years of trying, I hit a low point. And then when my sister got pregnant with her sixth child, I practically lost it. It just didn't seem fair. I would think about all the babies born to families who already had six, eight, or ten children. I would think about babies born addicted to drugs because their mothers used during pregnancy. I would see women at the grocery store who didn't have teeth … but they had three kids and another one on the way. I would wonder how, if they can't take care of their teeth, are they going to take care of these children?

I became very depressed at the thought of never having kids of my own. And all the triggers around me made it worse. I'd go to work and have to listen to a colleague complain about all the baby weight she was gaining. I'd look at social media, and post after post was filled with pictures of fetal ultrasounds and newborns. I'd go to family dinners, and everybody was oohing and aahing over the new baby. And in the middle of all this, I would try to keep a smile on my face … while on the inside, I felt like I was dying. I'd usually hold it together long enough to make it through whatever situation I was in, then I'd cry all the way home and usually the rest of the day.

At that point, I started going to counseling. My therapist taught me some important lessons about self-care and boundaries. She told me that self-preservation was key. That was hard to accept because I've always put others before myself. But, in order to get through this thing, I made the decision to put a boundary between myself and anything related to babies. I couldn't avoid every situation, but many of them

I could. I stopped volunteering in our church nursery. I stopped using social media. And for a while, I chose to stay home whenever the family gathered for various holidays and celebrations. This really helped in a way because I didn't have to be around all the oohing and aahing over the new baby, but it hurt me in another way that I didn't anticipate. My family thought I was being selfish. They thought I wasn't acting like a Christian. They thought my therapist was a quack. They thought I was tearing the family apart. And they unloaded all this on my husband. Lucky for me, they never told me directly how they felt. But they took every opportunity they could to tell him.

Thankfully, my husband was very supportive. He listened when I needed to vent and held me when I cried and tried to defend me when he could. But I felt so bad for him because he was caught in the middle. He loved me. He felt the same pain I did. But he loved them, too. Ultimately, he took my side, but it wasn't without consequences. We got the cold shoulder much of the time. When there was communication, we got snide remarks. When there were events we did feel like we could attend, we weren't invited or flat out were asked not to come. And we were talked about. A lot. This lasted for years. I'm so fortunate my husband supported me because I know it could have gone the other way. He could have pushed me to get over it so we didn't have to deal with the drama. But he's always been my number one cheerleader and fan, the only one who truly stood by me through it all. I hate that he was caught in the middle. He never complained once. But sometimes I wonder if he ever felt resentful. Sometimes he says he wishes we could go back to the way life was before infertility. I wish we could, too, because nothing will ever be the same again. Not for us. And not definitely not for our family.

Social Media

Another type of friend in our society today is the social media friend. Social media is one of the primary ways for people to connect with each other in our world. While social media can serve as a source of information and social support for those suffering from infertility (Sormunen et al., 2020), it's impossible to look at social media without being inundated with posts about positive pregnancy tests, ultrasounds, gender reveals, baby showers, and birth announcements. While social media may be an important way to stay connected with others, these triggers can induce hurt and pain and serve as reminders of trauma related to infertility and reproductive loss. Those suffering from infertility may need to avoid social media if it has a negative impact on their emotional well-being. You may want to discuss with clients how social media impacts them so they can make informed decisions about when and whether to use it. And if they are unable to keep up with friends because of a Facebook fast, you can explore with them ways to make social connections in other meaningful ways.

In this section, we explored the social impact of infertility related to friends and family. We looked at how hurtful comments, a lack of understanding and empathy, and even social media can negatively impact the hero's support system and emotional well-being. Now let's explore another important relational aspect, the relationship with faith.

RELATIONSHIP WITH FAITH

One function of spirituality is the meaning and purpose to life it can give. In some instances, faith, spirituality, or the existential self can play a role in one's desire to become a parent. Some people may feel a call to action to make the world a better place or simply want a meaningful way to give back a little of what was given to them. Some, however, believe they have a spiritual calling to reproduce. Many people struggling with infertility experience great frustration when they can't fulfill this higher-level spiritual purpose. If they have a strong commitment to a particular faith system or a relationship with a higher power, they may encounter additional spiritual crises.

Spiritual beliefs often provide a sense of purpose and comfort in adversity (Roudsari et al., 2009). For some, their personal belief system is a foundational part of who they are. What happens then when one's circumstances are at odds with their beliefs? A crisis of faith can occur. For example, Christians often rely on the Bible for guidance. In Genesis 1:28 of the Bible, humans are directed to be fruitful and multiply (King James Version, 1769/2022). What does this mean for someone who takes this command literally but is then unable to conceive? In addition, many faith systems encourage prayer and supplication when making requests from their higher power. What does it mean for a person who prays continually for children, but those requests aren't granted? What does that say about God as the giver of life? Or their relationship with God? What does that say about faith and prayer? What does it mean when a higher power who is loving and kind allows people to go through a trial like infertility that causes so much heartache and pain? For those whose faith system involves a personal relationship with their higher power, this relationship may even be negatively impacted. Some may get angry with their higher power and even turn away from their faith as a result.

Another potential crisis may occur when spiritual beliefs and practices, once a source of strength and comfort, become a source of pain. Consider those who attend church as part of organized religion. Going to church may usually be comforting and encouraging, but on Mother's Day and Father's Day, many churches have baby dedications or deliver sermons about parenthood that can trigger negative emotions for those experiencing infertility. Finding a place to fit in may also be a challenge because small group classes composed of people similar in age to the hero may be filled with couples who have babies or are expecting. These experiences may lead those suffering from infertility to avoid certain gatherings that induce heartache or maybe even lead them to avoid organized religion altogether.

Faith systems can cause turmoil in other ways. Religious beliefs and clergy have largely influenced the way we view issues such as marriage, divorce, birth, and death. When assisted reproductive technologies were developed in the late 20th century, they were welcomed by some religions, but attacked by others (Sallam & Sallam, 2016). Today, assisted reproduction is accepted in most forms by Buddhists, Hindus, Jews, Protestants, Coptic Christians, Anglicans, and Sunni Muslims, while it remains unacceptable for Roman Catholics. And while many religions accept assisted reproduction in most forms, others, such as Orthodox Jews, Sunni Muslims, and Chinese Confucianists do not accept third-party involvement such as embryo donation (Sallam & Sallam, 2016).

As helping professionals, you may encounter clients, supervisees, or students who have strong desires to pursue alternative routes to parenthood that conflict with their religion's stance on assisted reproduction. This could lead to a dissonance between fulfilling hopes and dreams and loyalty to the traditions of their faith system. It is imperative to take time to explore these relationships and conflicts with faith. This can assist you with identifying problem areas such as spiritual crises and belief conflicts. In addition, remember to explore spiritual beliefs as opportunities for hope and healing because faith is such a foundational part of many people's lives.

MARIA'S STORY

My husband and I married in 2004 when I was 23 years old. He was ten years older and had an eight-year-old son from a previous marriage. I had been told as a teenager that I probably had polycystic ovarian syndrome, but it was never confirmed with anything other than an ultrasound. I was thin, active, and a healthy young woman. I never dreamed I would have trouble becoming pregnant! In 2005 I stopped taking birth control because of some side effects (mood swings) I was experiencing. We had decided to go ahead and start trying, foolishly assuming that I would quickly become pregnant. I was so excited! However, after a year of being off of birth control, I never became pregnant. My primary care physician referred me to one of the top specialists in our city. I was so hopeful that he would be our ally. At my first appointment, he sat and listened to me talk – about the polycystic ovarian syndrome, my irregular periods, and not becoming pregnant. I will never forget his response. He told me with utter confidence that I would never be able to get pregnant without his help.

I was devastated. As a Christian, I felt like he was playing God and taking too much credit. I never went back to him. My wonderful primary care physician referred me to another fertility specialist. He was compassionate and understanding and worked to properly diagnose me and treat my problems. After a hysterogram, blood work, ultrasounds, and exams, he confirmed I do have polycystic ovarian syndrome and proceeded to treat my condition with an ultra-low-carb diet. Even though I was already thin, I lost 20 pounds with a baby as my hope and motivation. I felt amazing and was so excited. We then went through three rounds of Letrozole and Clomid injections over a period of four months. Despite our prayers, our best efforts, and a strict intimacy schedule, we never became pregnant. The doctor offered to progress to hormone injections, but I did not have peace and took a month off before we made a decision. The holidays passed, we continued remodeling our home, and then my husband lost his job. At that point I saw God's sovereignty in us not becoming pregnant three months prior.

My husband found a new job, we moved back into our home, and we enjoyed a lovely spring as a family of three while I continued to eat a low-carb diet. In May 2007, I discovered I was pregnant! All on our own! We were thrilled and so thankful for the answered prayer. The past two years had been long, lonely years filled with questions, tears, and uncomfortable medical procedures. I questioned God's plans and purposes for my life and wondered why others could have children and I could not.

Our daughter was born in January 2008. Her older brother was 12, and he was thrilled to have a baby sister. I hoped for more kids, but my husband and I could not quite agree on that. I went back on hormonal birth control, thinking that was a solution to my issues. Three years later we moved to a new state, and my prescription ran out. I had not yet had time to find a new doctor and warned my husband of the lack of birth control. We both were nonchalant about it since it had taken years to conceive our daughter. Well, surprise - within one month I became pregnant with our son. We were blown away! I struggled with the side effects from the mini pill while breastfeeding and stopped taking it. Shortly after our son's first birthday I found out I was pregnant with another daughter. I was so surprised! She started sleeping through the night at ten weeks, and within two months I became pregnant with our youngest daughter. I quickly told my husband we were done, and something had to change.

Our fertility journey is a story of God's sovereignty. Doctors can make promises or boast claims, but ultimately, they could not create the outcomes we wanted. Our timing looked different than we would have liked, but our family is now complete (despite my children's requests to add another boy!). We are so thankful. All our five children are miracles in their own right, and I am so thankful our first specialist was wrong when he told me I could never have children without his help!

RELATIONSHIP WITH SELF

For those experiencing infertility, perhaps one of the most difficult relationships to cope with is the relationship with the self. We already outlined the psychological impacts of infertility in Chapter 3, however, we do want to touch on it briefly again in this section because of the close connection that exists between psychological well-being and a sense of self which is essential for the hero in her journey.

One common response for our hero is self-blame and doubt. While self-blame and doubt may have been present prior to an infertility diagnosis, these feelings can intensify. Sufferers may experience shame related to not being able to pass on the family name or genetic code. They may experience a loss of identity when the only thing they've ever dreamed about is being a parent, and it doesn't happen. They may blame themselves for being defective or for not trying hard enough. Self-loathing may occur when the hero's body does not function the way it's intended. And many sufferers have worked hard at and been successful at most things they've tried in life, but now they feel like failures because this is one thing they just can't make happen, no matter how hard they try.

Some who set boundaries for their own emotional well-being may feel guilty for not attending family gatherings or for feeling jealous. The hurtful comments from others just make it all worse. "I can't believe he's acting like this," "She's not the person I thought she was," and "She should be over this by now" add to the guilt. Sufferers may take these comments personally and get angry with themselves for not being able to just get over it. One woman stated, "I'm broken. I internalized it. It was about me, it was how I lacked a certain drive, or certain faith, or something that everybody else seems to have that I didn't" (McBain & Reeves, 2019, p.160). Coming to terms with self in the face of infertility may be one of the biggest challenges of all.

CONCLUSION

We've come to the end of Part One of the book. Our hero has experienced a call to adventure that will leave her forever changed. Although she may wish to, she cannot avoid the journey, but where does she go from here? Her biological, psychological, and social struggles set the stage for additional conflicts. In Part Two of this book, we explore the road of trials as the hero embarks on the quest. While the challenges of infertility have long been considered a female problem, the dilemma also includes other populations. In Part Two, we delve deeper into other groups who experience unique struggles related to infertility. These include those suffering from age-related infertility, those with non-age-related infertility, those who struggle with femininity and the social implications of infertility, men, those seeking nontraditional ways to conceive, and those coming from a variety of cultural backgrounds. We will also explore the cultural and interpersonal ramifications of pursuing a nontraditional pregnancy. Grab some popcorn and a blanket. Our adventure continues. And our hero awaits.

REFERENCES

Andrews, F.M., Abbey, A., & Halman, L.J. (1991). Stress from infertility, marriage factors, and subjective well-being of wives and husbands. *Journal of Health and Social Behavior*, *32*(3), 238–253. 10.2307/2136806

Hostinar, C. E. & Gunnar, M.R. (2015). Social support can buffer against stress and shape brain activity. *AJOB Neuroscience*, *6*(3), 34–42. 10.1080/21507740. 2015.1047054

Javaid, B., Ajmal, R., Ahmad, U., Rashed, A.A., Khan, A.B., Batool, H., Zainab, F., & Safdar (2022). Marital dissatisfaction and depression: A comparative study among infertile couples of Punjab. *Pakistan Journal of Medical and Health Sciences*, *16*(7), 243–244. 10.53350/pjmhs22167243

King James Bible. (2022). King James Bible Online. https://www.kingjamesbible online.org/ (Original work published 1769)

Kjaer, T., Albieri, V., Jensen, A., Kjaer, S.K., Johansen, C., & Dalton, S.O. (2014). Divorce or end of cohabitation among Danish women evaluated for fertility problems. *Acta Obsetricia et Gynecologica Scandinavica*, *93*(3), 269–276. 10.1111/aogs.12317

McBain, T. D., & Reeves, P. (2019). Women's experience of infertility and disenfranchised grief. *The Family Journal*, *27*(2), 156–166. 10.1177/1066480719833418

Roudsari, R.L., Allan, H.T., & Smith, A.L. (2009). Looking at infertility through the lens of religion and spirituality: A review of the literature. *Human Fertility*, *10*(3), 141–149. 10.1080/14647270601182677

Sallam, H.N., & Sallam, N.H. (2016). Religious aspects of assisted reproduction. *Facts, Views, and Vision in ObGyn*, *8*(1), 33–48.

Sormunen, T., Karlgren, K., Aanesen, A., Fossum, B., & Westerboth, M. (2020). The role of social media for persons affected by infertility. *BMC Women's Health*, *20*(12), 1–8. 10.1186/s12905-020-00964-0

Tao, P., Coates, R., & Maycock, B. (2011). The impact of infertility on sexuality: A literature review. *Australasian Medical Journal*, *4*(11), 620–627.

Wu, A.K. (2014). Out-of-pocet fertility patient expense: Data from a multicenter prospective infertility cohort. *Journal of Urology*, *191*(2), 427–432. 10.1016/j.juro.2013.08.083

PART TWO

Who Suffers from Infertility?

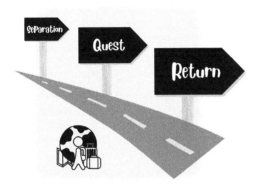

DOI: 10.4324/9781003336402-7

CHAPTER FIVE

Aging and Infertility

TICK, TICK, TICK … Is That My
Biological Clock?

Too old? Really?

Films, TV shows, popular music, and even Tik Tok reels depict the often humorous impasse, the image of the eager female and hesitant male partner in a sort of tussle over commitment. This tug of war is excellent fodder for humor, but the cautionary tale often turns out to be true. Women dating in their 20s and 30s, attuned to their limited time to become mothers, put themselves in a sort of dating pressure cooker, a modern-day Instapot.

Women's biology binds them to a window of time in which conceiving a child is possible. A woman's peak fertility years span from the late teens to the mid-20s. As the aging process continues, fertility declines slowly at first, then drops precipitously around the age of 35 (American College of Obstetricians and Gynecologists, 2020). After age 40, complications such as preeclampsia significantly increase in addition to birth complications including miscarriage, stillbirth, and increased risk of preterm birth. As a woman ages, natural conception, or even assisted conception, becomes increasingly challenging. Our hero may be getting older and experiencing the consequences associated with fertility and aging.

As aging women struggle with the physical, emotional, and hormonal changes associated with maturing, these issues are amplified for those seeking to conceive. The fertility timeline often conflicts with necessary precursors to child-bearing, such as finding a partner and establishing professional and financial stability. We've been acutely aware of the parts necessary for conception since middle school health class. Those who inevitably sat through these mortifying educational experiences are aware of how and when conception can occur. While pursuing education, networking, and acquiring professional accolades, women

DOI: 10.4324/9781003336402-8

are navigating their chosen professional environment, while often simultaneously struggling with their journey to motherhood.

While declining a promise ring from a high school suitor or rebuffing the proposal of their college beau, these women were likely at the time unaware of the biological consequences associated with their decision to delay parenthood. As a result of these decisions, they may have trouble conceiving or be unable to conceive, coupled with existential reflection and regrets. If conception does occur among older women, it is coupled with increased possibilities of high-risk pregnancies and birth defects. For example, the likelihood of Down Syndrome increases substantially from 1 in 1,480 at age 20 to 1 in 35 at age 45 (American College of Obstetricians and Gynecologists, 2020).

These often private fertility struggles are exacerbated by the seemingly constant parade of celebrations surrounding peers' pregnancies and rituals such as baby showers and selecting names. In Part One, we explored the biological, psychological, and social impacts of infertility. Throughout Part Two, we will examine various people groups who encounter unique struggles related to the condition. Chapter 5 focuses on the unique experiences of women facing age-related infertility. These include having a limited window for conception, cultural and societal influences, physical limitations, social support and intimate relationship difficulties, and financial considerations.

A LIMITED WINDOW

Lucille Ball was credited with saying that "the secret to staying young is to live honestly, eat slowly, and lie about your age" (Ball, n.d.). Ah, to be young. For some women, youth is synonymous with beauty and desirability; it also parallels peak fertility and childbearing years. With youth comes privilege: energy, health, societal admiration, and even aspiration. Society says women aspire to be young. However, unlike other tenets of privilege, youth is fleeting. In addition to the societal obsession with the physical attributes of youth, being younger increases the likelihood of conception, with fewer risks of complications for a woman or her unborn child. In many ways, cultural norms and gender roles have evolved and grown incongruous with a woman's biological window of fertility.

Although the onset of the menstrual period is decreasing (Martinez, 2020), a woman's ability to conceive parallels her first menstrual period, which on average begins as young as 11 or 12. This is in stark contrast to the cultural norms of the age of marriage and childbearing in the United States. Fortunately, our better understanding of child development limits young adolescents from legally marrying. Most states allow legal marriage over the age of 15 with parental consent. Massachusetts is the outlier, permitting marriage at the age of 12 until only recently when an amendment that prohibited the marriage of minors became effective (Mass. General Laws c.207 § 7, 2022). By the time a woman can legally marry and care autonomously for a child, she is ten years into the 30- to 40-year window during which conception and the birth of a child are even possible. Perhaps our hero's call to action was a slower, more multi-faceted one, peppered with consideration for a variety of life choices, delaying her journey. Maybe she is the product of an archaic intersection of biology, inter-personal, and societal norms in her drive toward motherhood.

CULTURAL AND SOCIETAL INFLUENCES

The legal regulation of teenage marriage reflects societal shifts in America and other first-world countries. Although inequities in positions of power and earning potential remain, women are generally viewed as equals, rather than girls ush-ered from their primary family to a husband's home. Feminism and advance-ments in women's rights have substantially broadened women's options. Although afforded the opportunity to focus on motherhood and more traditional roles, during the 20th century other opportunities have become feasible for women. Opportunities for education and career advancement coupled with desires for motherhood and caregiving can both liberate and limit women. While women's rights have advanced substantially, our biological clocks have not caught up. This leaves women who have prioritized self-exploration and other pursuits with the physical and emotional ramifications of postponing mother-hood. For the helping professional, these factors must be integrated into our interactions, gauging our hero's understanding and feelings associated with the factors that placed her in the predicament of age-related infertility.

PHYSICAL COMPLICATIONS

The physical risks associated with pursuing pregnancy later in life are present not only for the mother but potentially the child. This brings another set of issues to navigate. The results of one study identified significant increases in maternal mortality rates for older women (Hoyert, 2022). In the year 2020, mortality rates for women under age 25 were 13.8 deaths per 100,000 live births. For those aged 25–39, the rate was 22.8, and for those aged 40 and older, the rate was 107.9. These statistics indicate that the rate of maternal mortality for women over 40 years of age was over 7.8 times that of women under 25. Beyond the risks to the mother, a multitude of threats exist for the child. Risks of miscarriage, stillbirth, and infant mortality are correlated with maternal age beyond 35 (Correa-de-Araujo & Yoon, 2022). The most difficult decision our hero may make could be related to whether to continue a pregnancy following the detection of birth defects or limited life expectancy for the fetus. Medical advancements allow insight into the chromosomal characteristics of a fetus in early months, with results showing the risk of babies having Down Syndrome jumping from 1 in 1,480 at age 20 to 1 in 35 at age 45 (American College of Obstetricians and Gynecologists, 2020). Similar correlations are found between Trisomy 13 and 18 – chromosomal conditions which are characterized by triads rather than dyads on certain chromosomes – and increased maternal age, while non-chromosomal defects, such as heart and soft palate deformities, are also linked to aging mothers (Witters et al., 2011).

As helping professionals, you should know that this double bind presents difficult, sometimes impossible, decisions for women who have postponed their role as a mother, leaving them to grapple with the physical limitations and risks associated with delayed pregnancy. A woman taking advantage of the opportunities afforded to her by years of crusading is regaled for her accomplishments while simultaneously bound by the constraints that aging places on her ability to enter the more traditional role of motherhood. As time and energy are invested in furthering a woman's personal and professional identity, she loses footing in her physical ability to conceive and carry to full-term a healthy child.

SOCIAL SUPPORTS AND INTIMATE RELATIONSHIP DIFFICULTIES

In addition to the physical limitations and risks of delayed pregnancy, women who postpone conception are frequently faced with changing interactions with their social support systems and peer networks. Often, those who delay parenthood experience shifts in their social interactions as others choose to pursue parenthood. While traditional baby showers became popularized in the United States in the 1940s and 50s following the baby boom, today's celebrations often go far beyond that. Secular celebrations often include a baby reveal, gender reveal, shower, and sip and see coupled with baby namings. Bris and baptisms immediately following the birth of a child offer their own celebrations. The value of these events cannot be understated. For the parent, child, and community, they are established rites of passage. For those struggling with infertility, however, participation in these events can create a painful double bind.

These shifts in social interactions may occur gradually or seemingly all at once. For those who postpone motherhood, feelings of isolation may increase as the distance between friends may arise over the changing demographics (Kiesswetter et al., 2020). Social encounters may shift from individual outings and couples' dinner dates to playdates or other child-centric activities. For those who have either postponed parenthood or are facing the challenges of infertility, these shifts in social worlds can be emotionally charged and negatively impact life satisfaction.

In addition to difficulties with social support networks, our hero often faces challenges related to intimate partner relationships. Playwright George Bernard Shaw said, "It is a woman's business to get married as soon as possible and a man's to keep unmarried as long as he can" (2017). To conceive within one's fertile window, one typically needs a partner. Although the concept of the old maid has become less overtly expressed, the pressure to couple prior to conceiving remains. Often, women desire a suitable partner with whom to embark upon this journey. Again, settling down into a traditional, if not obsolete, two-parent American family falls into the general societal expectations of a woman (Brunch & Newman, 2018). Ironically, as women take advantage of opportunities for education and career advancement and pursue other options, the ability to meet a partner often lessens. This results in seeking partnerships through non-organic means, such as online dating or dating apps, which bring about their own set of difficulties. Limitations associated with finding a potential partner were most recently amplified by the onset of a global pandemic in 2020 when physical contact with those outside of one's bubble was often prohibited by law.

In addition to the pursuit of education during peak fertility years, placing relationships on the back burner while pursuing education and career impacts our hero's ability to find a partner. Brunch and Newman (2018) found that not only did female attractiveness to male partners on dating apps decrease with age, but an inverse correlation between education and attractiveness existed as well. This was true for women, but the researchers found the opposite results for men. Older, well-educated women were less likely to be seen as attractive, which poses a consequence for starting and maintaining relationships – a natural precursor to motherhood. By the age of 45, a woman's likelihood of conceiving naturally does not exceed 3% or 4%. If a woman can conceive, the likelihood of a healthy delivery substantially decreases. In addition, the likelihood of having a baby with birth defects or health issues substantially increases.

Assuming a woman can find a partner and give birth to a child, another difficult decision arises. Will she work or not? Women make up a large portion of the workforce, and the gender wage gap has been found to be directly related to the responsibilities of parenthood remaining with the mother instead of the father. Women are again caught between professional goals and identity and the drive to start a family. Ideally, women and men seek and maintain a career that not only creates financial independence and success but also merges with their professional and personal identities. A woman may be presented with the decision to either maintain that professional identity, relinquish it to be fully present in motherhood, or find some middle ground.

The concept of having it all is quickly eliminated because, although career and motherhood can occur simultaneously, the balance is often precarious and interspersed with compromises affecting both roles.

FINANCIAL CONSIDERATIONS

The financial freedom to choose between the option to work or stay home with a child is one only afforded to a small portion of privileged mothers. The expenses associated with having and raising a child are prohibitive, and often the choice to stay home is not a viable option for a mother as her earnings are necessary to maintain the household. Often, debt accrued to cover fertility treatments can also significantly impact a woman's choice to enter the workforce or not. For those in more ideal situations, the cost-benefit analysis of comparing childcare costs to salary and benefits is a common predictor of decisions. The awareness of the financial responsibility associated with having children can further postpone the decision and consequently result in difficulty in doing so.

CONCLUSION

As peers shift focus to a child-centric world, the hero's often private struggle with infertility seeps into the entire landscape of her life and affects religious, cultural, social, financial, and even professional roles. While feminist leaders such as Sheryl Sandberg encourage women to lean in and place career aspirations beyond all else (2013), this logic flies in the face of what we know about fertility and the aging process. Are we to lean in professionally, assuming relationships and children will simply fall into place, or place our proverbial eggs in the family basket, dedicating precious time, money, and energy to motherhood? These decisions can be challenging to navigate, resulting in substantial emotional distress for our hero.

REFERENCES

American College of Obstetricians and Gynecologists. (2020). *Having a baby after age 35: How Aging Affects Fertility and Pregnancy*. https://www.acog.org/womens-health/faqs/having-a-baby-after-age-35-how-aging-affects-fertility-and-pregnancy

Ball, L. (n.d.). *Lucille Ball Quote. Libquotes*. https://libquotes.com/lucille-ball/quote/lbb9o1a

Brunch, E. E., & Newman, M. E. J. (2018). Aspirational pursuit of mates in online dating markets. *Science Advances*, *4*(8). https://www.science.org/doi/10.1126/sciadv.aap9815

Correa-de-Araujo, R. & Yoon, S.S. (2022). Clinical outcomes in high-risk pregnancies due to advanced maternal age. *Journal of Women's Health (Larchmt)*, *30*(2), 160–167. 10.1089/jwh.2020.8860

Hoyert, D.L. (2022). *Maternal Mortality Rates in the United States, 2020*. National Center for Health Statistics. 10.15620/cdc:113967

Kiesswetter, M., Marsoner, H., Luehwink, A., Fistarol, M., Mahlknecht, A., & Duschek, S. (2020). Impairments in life satisfaction in infertility: Associations with perceived stress, affectivity, partnership quality, social support and the desire to have a child. *Behavioral Medicine*, *46*(2), 130–141. 10.1080/08964289.201 8.1564897

Martinez, G. M. (2020). Trends and patterns in menarche in the United States: 1995 through 2013–2017. *National Health Statistics Reports*, 146, 1–12.

Mass. General Laws c.207 § 7 (2022).

Sandberg, S. (2013). *Lean in: Women, work, and the will to lead* (First edition.). Alfred A. Knopf.

Shaw, G. B. (2017). *Bernard Shaw's Marriages and Misalliance*s. Palgrave Macmillan.

Witters, G., Van Robays, J., Willekes, C., Coumans, A., Peeters, H., Gyselaers, W., & Fryns, J. P. (2011). Trisomy 13, 18, 21, Triploidy and Turner syndrome: the 5T's. Look at the hands. *Facts, Views & Vision in ObGyn*, *3*(1), 15–21.

CHAPTER SIX

Non-Age-Related Infertility

I'm Still a Spring Chicken, So Where Are My Chicks?

"Wait … I'm still young, right?"

"I thought I had more time!"

Or the dreaded, "My mother was right, I should've settled down earlier."

Thoughts like these often fill the inner monologue of young women unsuccessfully trying to have children. With the realization that non-age-related infertility is a factor, women often find themselves surprised and overwhelmed with the possibilities that lie ahead. While age is the primary predictor of fertility among women, it does not account for all difficulties in conceiving and delivering a healthy baby. This population, who suffers from non-age-related infertility, those not afforded the biological freedom to choose parenthood during their fertility window, requires unique support. Congenital, medical, or environmental issues can create barriers to our hero's attempts to become a mother. She may also grapple with mental health issues associated with this journey, or be part of marginalized groups for whom natural conception is impossible. We will explore these issues throughout this chapter.

WHAT IS NON-AGE-RELATED INFERTILITY?

If I'm not too old, what's the problem? One-third of infertility issues are attributed to the male reproductive system, one-third attributed to the female reproductive system, and one-third is attributed to a combination of the two or an unidentified

DOI: 10.4324/9781003336402-9

issue (Cleveland Clinic, 2020). This distinction of the root of infertility, while seemingly irrelevant, is important for both medical professionals and helping professionals. The specifics of infertility epidemiology and prognosis are accompanied by a distinct set of emotional and contextual difficulties. Throughout Chapter 6, we will specifically address female infertility that is unrelated to aging (non-age-related female infertility).

TYPES OF NON-AGE-RELATED INFERTILITY

Although age is the primary factor in a woman's fertility (American College of Obstetricians and Gynecologists, 2020), a woman's ability to conceive may be adversely impacted by a variety of issues. These issues may include but not be limited to illness, injury, congenital problems, reproductive health concerns, use of prescription medication, mental health disorders, and hormonal disturbances. In some instances, women may attempt to conceive later and find that age compounds the presence of these factors, adding layers of difficulty to the client's journey. Some women know from a young age that pregnancy may be difficult for them, but many others remain blissfully ignorant of health complications that could interfere with fertility until they find themselves with a negative pregnancy test month after month of attempting to conceive.

The congenital and environmental barriers to pregnancy experienced by young heterosexual women in traditional male/female relationships are difficult but constitute only a fraction of those struggling with infertility. Of all marital statuses, 9.2% of females ages 15–29 and 22.2% of females ages 30–39 reported the inability to conceive or the inability to remain pregnant, making this experience relatively common (Centers for Disease Control and Prevention, 2021). However, it is important to acknowledge non-age-related, which infertility occurs within the context of a variety of relationships, both traditional heterosexual and alternative partnerships. Individuals in homosexual relationships experience biological and social barriers to conception independent of age. These biological difficulties are amplified by societal and financial hurdles limiting options for this population.

HOW IS THIS DIFFERENT FROM OTHER KINDS OF INFERTILITY?

I'm young, and I'm healthy. Why can't I conceive? While physiological limitations associated with age-related infertility are relatively well understood, individual non-age-related infertility limitations often present an invisible struggle. One's chronological age is generally apparent. People can usually guess how old another individual is with some accuracy. Individual and societal assumptions are that if you aren't too old, then the ability to successfully conceive should be relatively uncomplicated. Therefore, infertility problems for this population often result in a unique struggle accompanied by a lack of social and societal acknowledgment and support. This struggle is often steeped in grief, often disenfranchised grief (Doka, 1989, 1999, 2002), at each stage of fertility loss.

When that window to conceive is truncated or not viable at all, women often sense that their bodies have betrayed them and endure the consequences. It is at this point that the confluence of femininity and purpose tied to a woman's ability to reproduce occurs. A woman suffering from non-age-related infertility may face existential questions about purpose, fertility, and identity. Although your role as helping professionals is not to diagnose or treat medical issues associated with difficulty conceiving, it is imperative that we are aware of the factors which contribute to the difficulties in our clients' fertility journeys.

CONGENITAL ISSUES IMPACTING INFERTILITY

Congenital issues are those that have existed since birth, occurring during pre-natal or early fetal development (World Health Organization, 2022). These health problems can be far-reaching and impact the hero throughout her life. In 2017, the U.S. Department of Health and Human Services reported that the following congenital health conditions are directly related to an inability to conceive: auto-immune disorders, endocrine issues, and structural malformation of the repro-ductive organs. At birth, women have their entire reproductive system, consisting of a uterus, fallopian tubes, and ovaries; damage or malformation of these can limit a woman's fertility at birth. Other congenital issues, such as malformation of non-secondary sex characteristics, are established during fetal development, and she is born with all the eggs she will ever have (Woodruff, 2008).

In some cases, congenital female reproductive issues are often attributed to some combination of genetic and environmental factors. While fertility is often not at the forefront of a woman's periphery until she comes of childbearing age, congenital issues related to infertility may be at the root of our hero's problem. Essentially, some components of a woman's ability to become a mother may be determined prior to her own birth. This information may bring our hero to an existential crisis, mourning the fact that she was never able to have children.

ENVIRONMENTAL IMPACTS ON FERTILITY

In addition to the congenital health-related limitations identified previously, contextual experiences can create barriers to conception as a woman ages, resulting in non-age-related infertility. Women who are born with the biological capability to have children may experience illness, injury, or sexual identity issues that limit their likelihood of natural conception and the birth of a healthy baby. Infections associated with the acquisition of sexually transmitted infections such as gonorrhea and chlamydia may result in pelvic inflammatory disease. If left untreated, pelvic inflammatory disease permanently mitigates a woman's ability to conceive (Centers for Disease Control, 2022b). A human papillomavirus infection accompanied by cervical lesions can also impede fertility (Centers for Disease Control, 2022c). Termination of an earlier pregnancy through either medical or surgical abortion, while long thought to impact the ability to conceive in the future, has been found to inhibit fertility in only rare cases (Virk et al., 2007). A difficult birth earlier in a woman's life may also lead to medical complications such as hemorrhage or infection, jeopardizing the mother's health at the time and potentially limiting her ability to have additional children.

MEDICAL IMPACTS ON FERTILITY

Most recently, a holistic approach to medicine has emphasized the interconnectedness between different systems in the human body. Medical issues associated with infertility include polycystic ovarian syndrome, heart disease, cancer, and sexually transmitted infections as well as complications associated with a previous pregnancy or abortion. Throughout this section, instead of identifying an ailment as an independent issue in the body, we will examine the system as a whole, exploring whether it is an acute issue or whether it may be indicative of a larger underlying issue. Although sometimes it is difficult to identify the primary issue from which infertility stems, it is important that we recognize the integrative nature of health and how these medical issues impact our clients.

Polycystic Ovarian Syndrome

Polycystic ovarian syndrome is the most common cause of female infertility and is a condition that causes women to ovulate irregularly, if at all (Centers for Disease Control and Prevention, 2022a). This disorder can also lead to increased levels of testosterone resulting in unpleasant side effects, such as increased acne and hair growth. Related to polycystic ovarian, it is a diminished ovarian response, another ovarian-related condition known to impact fertility, characterized by the ovaries holding fewer eggs than expected.

Heart Disease

In the early part of the 20th century, heart disease was associated more with older men; however, today heart disease remains the leading cause of death among women (Centers for Disease Control and Prevention, 2022d). Although symptoms associated with heart disease typically have a later onset among females than men (age 65+) and generally occur post-menopause, connections between heart disease and infertility exist. According to a 2017 study, surmounting evidence suggests that heart problems are associated with specific infertility conditions such as ovarian disease, polycystic ovarian syndrome, endometriosis, and thyroid dysfunction (Verit et al., 2017). Again, all of these are known to negatively impact reproductive viability.

Cancer

Although we have yet to identify a cure for cancer, substantial advancements in the treatment of cancer have occurred over the past several decades. A cancer diagnosis results in profound physical and emotional difficulties; for those who still hope to become parents, the diagnosis may seem insurmountable. The ability of a woman to conceive following cancer diagnosis and treatment is contingent upon many variables, but the most influential seems to be the type of treatment she receives. According to the American Cancer Society (2020), this type of cancer is highly relevant to a subsequent diagnosis of infertility. Non-age-related fertility complications directly related to a cancer diagnosis may include uterine, ovarian, or thyroid. In some instances, treatment for cancer can jeopardize infertility (Duffy & Allen, 2009). Treatment options such as radiation (specifically occurring near the pelvis or brain), chemotherapy, and hormone treatment may result in decreased fertility among women. While managing difficult diagnoses and health issues associated with cancer, women and their partners also may face difficult decisions about future avenues to fertility such as egg retrieval and freezing eggs.

KELLY'S STORY

I was diagnosed with a rare brain tumor in 2006. I was attending my first year of college at the University of Tennessee at Chattanooga (UTC). The tumor was rare they said, common in young boys. I was 19. Each neurosurgeon told me the same thing … .the surgery could leave me blind, and I may never be able to have kids. Fast forward to 2013 when I met the man of my dreams and married in 2014. We tried on our own before confirming what the doctors said. We made an appointment with the local reproductive endocrinologist. We followed his protocol, spent thousands of dollars on tests and procedures, and finally began the intrauterine insemination process. We tried this two times. Each time was a failure and a reminder of the possibility of never becoming pregnant and never having kids. This led us to another fertility specialist and started our journey of in vitro fertilization. More money and more tests, but this time we were hopeful.

The egg retrieval went well! We had 11 total, and three made it to the final stage. We returned to Nashville for the embryo transfer to later find out we were pregnant! Then we began daily injections to hopefully stay pregnant. The story gets better. My brain surgery in Nashville was May 4th, and after making a complete circle and replacing a bad memory with a good (IVF in Nashville), our beautiful daughter was born in May! May is a very special month for us! We also had a beautiful baby boy born by IVF the following July.

Sexually Transmitted Infections

According to the Centers for Disease Control (2022c), despite the presence of a global pandemic, 2.4 million cases of syphilis, gonorrhea, and chlamydia were reported in the past several years, with nearly one in five individuals in the United States infected at any given time. The physical symptoms associated with these infections are often dwarfed by the stigma of the diagnosis. Even the nomenclature change from sexually transmitted diseases to the less stigmatized term of sexually transmitted infections hints at an attempt at euphemism. Few disorders are coupled with a moral commentary, but sexually transmitted infections seem to check all the boxes. The presence of physical pain, emotional stress, and relational and interpersonal stressors following a diagnosis of a sexually transmitted infection are omnipotent and sometimes permanent. In many cases, they may have long-lasting ramifications, particularly for those trying to conceive following the diagnosis, another precursor for non-age-related infertility.

Specifically, two sexually transmitted infections, chlamydia, and gonorrhea, may result in pelvic inflammatory disease and tubal factor infertility in women (Tsevat et al., 2017). With approximately 1.5 million women in the United States labeled as infertile (Boivin et al., 2007), tubal factor infertility associated with pelvic inflammatory disease accounts for nearly 30% of these cases (Ross, 2013). This data emphasizes the strong correlation between sexually transmitted infections and the presence of subsequent fertility issues. As a helping professional, your work with individuals who have a history of or presence of this highly stigmatized diagnosis, compounded by the emotional and relational issues of infertility, requires a delicate approach.

Complications Associated with Earlier Pregnancy

"You should just be glad to have one child, some people can't even have that." "God must be telling you one is enough." These poorly delivered, yet well-intentioned messages fall from the mouths of parents, friends, and colleagues of our clients, landing with a thud of insensitivity. To those struggling with secondary infertility, unable to conceive following the birth of one or even multiple children, these statements are useless at best and inflammatory at worst. The idea that present circumstances should mitigate your desires to expand your family lacks logic and sensitivity.

Often, secondary infertility may be associated with complications from an earlier pregnancy, one either resulting in a healthy baby or termination by the mother. In the case where an earlier pregnancy ended in abortion, another layer of internal shame, integrated with potential religiously rooted guilt, may permeate the headspace of our hero. For those who have shared the decision to end the earlier pregnancy, statements from those with whom they surround themselves may be far more unkind than those listed at the beginning of this section.

Following the birth of an earlier child, medical conditions such as post-partum hemorrhage and hypovolemic shock have the highest likelihood of a post-birth hysterectomy and subsequent infertility (Zhang et al., 2017), yet the likelihood of a postpartum hysterectomy remains relatively low at .063% of the female population. The likelihood of limited fertility associated with complications of earlier pregnancy and/or delivery is not always as clear. In extreme cases, such as when a woman experiences a medical emergency like a postpartum hemorrhage, the decision about whether to have more children through natural means is made for her, compounding feelings of lacking agency over her own body. Other, less severe, complications following a prior birth often place our hero and her partner in a difficult situation when it comes to making medical decisions relevant to the ability to conceive. The couple may be faced with weighing the possibility of lifelong effects from issues related to high blood pressure, preeclampsia, gestational diabetes, and pre-term labor (U.S. Department of Health and Human Services, 2017) against her desire for more children.

You, the helping professional, may have struggled with or be close to someone who is unable to have a single healthy child. In these instances, you might need to bracket your biases. Countertransference is real, and often helping professionals are blind to it. Perhaps, deep down, you believe these clients should count themselves lucky to have been successful in their fertility journey at all. While it is human to experience our clients through our own lens, it is imperative that we are cognizant of these thoughts and emotions, keeping them separate from our interactions with clients. We must keep their experiences and perspectives at the forefront of the helping relationship.

Post-Abortion Infertility

Abortion is the medically or chemically induced ending of a pregnancy. Some women have elective abortions, and in some cases, the decision is made for them. Regardless of the mother's involvement in the decision-making process, abortion does have the potential to mitigate a woman's ability for future conception.

Since the legalization of medical abortions in 1973, the risk of complications to the mothers' health and the likelihood of future pregnancies decreased, with fewer than 1% of women requiring hospitalization following the completion of legal medical abortion (Upadhyay et al., 2018). This percentage is in stark contrast to the 13.2% of maternal deaths linked to abortions performed in countries where abortion is illegal (World Health Organization, 2021). In addition to factors related to the mother's general health, the likelihood of a woman having complications associated with fertility because of a previous abortion does occur but is very infrequent (Hogue, 1986). As the legalization of abortion varies now from state to state, the prospect of our client having an illegal and dangerous abortion is real. As helping professionals, working with those who face post-abortion infertility issues may test your personal beliefs. We are again tasked with deferring to our clients about their internal world including their thoughts, feelings, and if they hold a sense of responsibility or guilt associated with these decisions.

Throughout this section, we have explored the variety of medical issues which may contribute to or cause infertility or reproductive loss. While the developments of some of these issues are congenital and present at birth, others can arise with age, in addition to medical and surgical complications (Centers for Disease Control, 2022a). These medical issues are often unrelated to chronological age, conflating the difficulties of a medical diagnosis with the desire for parenthood now or in the future. The helping professional's awareness of these issues as well as associated struggles is imperative to the relationship and the process of healing.

MENTAL HEALTH AND FERTILITY

Infertility often results in emotional and mental health distress, but do mental health issues correlate to or even cause infertility? Research indicates that infertility is often the catalyst for emotional difficulties such as anxiety and depression; however, a debate exists over whether pre-existing mental health symptoms can have a negative impact on one's ability to conceive.

It appears that in addition to the mitigating factors that some physical health issues can have on one's ability to conceive, mental health issues may also have an effect. We will explore the correlation between mental health issues such as anxiety, depression, and disordered eating and our hero's ability to conceive.

Anxiety and Depression

Direct findings associated with formal diagnoses in the DSM-V-TR such as Generalized Anxiety Disorder or a Major Depressive Episode associated with non-age-related infertility are limited. A study by the American Society of Obstetrics found that a diagnosis of depression may create a decrease in the ability to conceive by nearly 40% (Nillni et al., 2016). Other studies indicate that successful treatment of anxiety and depression resulted in increased fertility rates among those diagnosed with infertility (Rooney & Domar, 2018; Sarrel & DeCherney, 1985). In some instances, a mental health issue may lead our hero to dysfunctional coping techniques (use of tobacco, alcohol, or drugs), the ramifications of which further limit her ability to conceive (Angelis et al., 2019).

Disordered Eating

Research indicates a direct relationship exists between infertility and bulimia, binge-eating disorder, and anorexia nervosa (Dağ & Dilbaz, 2015). These disorders often result in hormonal and metabolic dysfunction as well as extreme weight gain and loss, complicating one's ability to conceive. Disorders such as binge-eating disorder are likely to result in obesity. Women with a Body Mass Index greater than 30.0 are less likely to conceive, are at higher risk for miscarriage, and experience more complications during birth. Women who suffer from anorexia nervosa often have a BMI of less than 17.5, which can also result in difficulties with conception and the success of a healthy delivery (Chaer et al., 2020). Anorexia nervosa has also been linked to the condition known as functional hypothalamic amenorrhea, or the cessation of menstruation, which is caused by excessive exercise, weight loss, and/or stress (Centers for Disease Control 2022a; Podfigurna & Meczekalski, 2021). All these factors complicate the process of conception and pregnancy for the individual suffering from eating disorders.

As a helping professional, you are adept at diagnosis and intervention with those suffering from mental health disorders. While anxiety and depression may

NON-AGE-RELATED INFERTILITY

result in secondary physical issues such as hypertension or weight fluctuations, eating disorders have the most direct relationship to fertility concerns (Rooney & Domar, 2018). Mental health disorders are often exacerbated by, and at some times the cause of, non-age-related infertility.

For some women, pregnancy may result in the onset of mental health issues when they had been emotionally well prior to pregnancy. For example, post-partum depression impacts nearly one in seven mothers (Mughal et al., 2022). Attention to the possibility of a spectrum of emotional difficulties and mental health issues associated with pregnancy and birth again brings prospective mothers to a profoundly difficult decision. They are caught between weighing their desire to conceive with the risk of potential complications for their mental well-being. The helping professional must be prepared to walk with these heroes through this journey.

NON-HETEROSEXUAL COUPLES' INFERTILITY

Often, the nuances of defining same-sex or homosexual couples can feel like navigating a minefield. Medical and helping professionals are often paralyzed by anxiety and confusion related to how to address or define couples based on their current gender identity and sexual preference. The American Psychological Association (2014) came out with a sort of cheat sheet on definitions and appropriate terms to guide professionals in sensitivity regarding gender and sexual identity issues. To explore this group's infertility journey, we will define non-heterosexual couples as two individuals in an intimate partnership who share a gender identity.

Alternative Paths to Parenthood: Options for Non-Heteronormative Couples

Non-heterosexual couples are a marginalized group facing a multitude of societal barriers. Membership also automatically places them in the category of non-age-related infertility. Traditionally, conception and parenthood have been associated with a traditional male and female relationship, bringing a lack of acknowledgment of the unique challenges that homosexual couples face. For these individuals, awareness of their sexuality is followed by the realization that parenthood may be impossible. Later, hope may be rekindled with the ex-ploration of alternative means of parenthood for these couples. These couples are not infertile, by traditional definitions. The formal diagnosis of infertility used by most medical professionals and insurance companies is exclusionary to this population. The definition is based on sex between heterosexual partners, omitting this group altogether. Simply said, insurance won't cover assisted reproductive technology because these couples cannot meet diagnostic criteria for infertility. As a result, any insurance coverage to ease the financial burden of expensive procedures such as intrauterine insemination or in vitro fertilization is not possible for these couples.

ROBIN'S STORY

We had to plan every stage of wanting to become parents. It was weeks after marrying that planning our parenthood was in full swing. Since I didn't have the right plumbing, we needed to see what options were out there. There was no question that my wife was going to carry our child. We found a doctor that specializes in infertility and had a great success rate. We took out a $10,000 pension loan to pay for the out-of-network costs associated with the physician's services, and so our journey began.

Initially, we found a sperm donor. Next was all the testing. We both were required to have blood work performed. I found this endearing for myself personally since this was really the only biological contribution I felt like I was able to give during this entire process. My wife was immediately diagnosed with polycystic ovarian syndrome. Our doctor explained to us that although we would not be successful in getting pregnant through insemination, our insurance required us to try it three times before they would approve in vitro coverage. We were also faced with the decision and understanding of what "selective reduction" meant and coming to a place where if there were too many fertilized embryos, we had to decide which embryos to terminate, which was hard to imagine.

It took us about 18 months until we finally got pregnant. As a gay couple, during a time when gay marriage was not legal yet, I was placed into the sub-category of non-biological parent, which allowed the world to legally not recognize me as our children's parent. Gay marriage wasn't legalized in our state until three years after we had our civil union performed in Town Hall ... up until that point, the non-biological parent had to legally adopt his/her own children to ensure there was a legal document protecting the parent's right. It was an expensive process and demeaning. The adoption never took place in our first year of the twins' lives. Financially we couldn't afford it after spending thousands on medical bills, sperm purchase, and embryo storage. We had been together for seven years when the twins were born and were so happy that we, well I, didn't think it was necessary.

Our children had my last name and both of us were listed as the parents on the birth certificates.

My wife and I separated when the twins were about 18 months old. The scariest part in the split was the realization that I had no legal protection to see our children, and my soon to be ex-wife was exploiting my non-biological place in our children's lives. During our divorce and custody hearing, the presiding judge ruled that we were no different than a married couple. We dated, we got married, we got pregnant, and we had children. In the court's eyes, I was their equal parent and was awarded joint custody. I know this commentary is really based around the experiences I endured going through the infertility process, however, my journey was not like the one that most couples endure. I'm happy to see the world, both medically and socially, has changed for the better even in just the last ten years. I'm happy to report that despite the process, the court battles, and the painful realization of not being biologically connected to my twins, we maintain a strong relationship.

Our hero may not be a female, may not identify as female, and may not love a female, but she is on this journey just the same. Our hero's non-age-related infertility may be a biological construct of who she and her partner are. Nonetheless, they seek parenthood and experience the emotions associated with barriers to fulfilling this role similar to those in more traditional partnerships. As helping professionals, awareness of how non-hetero clients identify themselves and the barriers associated with belonging to a marginalized population are integral to assisting them through the challenges of non-age-related infertility.

CONCLUSION

We've seen that generally, women perceive they have a certain window in which conception is possible, and when this expectation is not met, these individuals embark on a difficult and often isolating journey. Women whose infertility is impacted by non-age-related factors experience a bevy of emotional and physiological difficulties. Physical health, congenital, medical, and environmental issues may adversely affect fertility despite a woman being in the prime of her childbearing years. Finally, mental health symptoms and diagnoses may also adversely impact her ability to conceive. An individual in a heterosexual relationship's ability to naturally conceive and deliver a healthy child is diminished by each of these issues, with varying likelihoods of success depending upon the intricacies of the circumstance. Despite the difficulties experienced by the heterosexual population, the issue of infertility is inherent in those who are seeking alternative paths to parenthood and who identify as non-heteronormative. This marginalized population may experience unique difficulties with conceiving and birthing a child in addition to the many societal barriers in place.

Throughout this chapter, we have identified a variety of non-age-related limitations associated with infertility. We also provided two vignettes illustrating how two women with different sexual identities and stories parallel one another. Both stories depict hope and disappointment, physical and emotional perseverance, and ultimately success. The successful achievement of the role of parent was obtainable for both individuals but may not be a viable outcome for all of those we are counseling. This disappointment carries another layer of discouragement and grief. In Chapter 7, we will explore how these emotional ramifications may also be amplified by contextual factors.

REFERENCES

American Cancer Society. (2020, February 6). *How cancer and cancer treatment can affect fertility in females*. https://www.cancer.org/treatment/treatments-and-side-effects/physical-side-effects/fertility-and-sexual-side-effects/fertility-and-women-with-cancer/how-cancer-treatments-affect-fertility.html

American College of Obstetricians and Gynecologists. (2020). *Having a baby after age 35: How aging affects fertility and pregnancy*. https://www.acog.org/womens-health/faqs/having-a-baby-after-age-35-how-aging-affects-fertility-and-pregnancy

American Psychological Association. (2014). *Answers to your questions about transgender people, gender identity, and gender expression*. [Pamphlet]. https://www.apa.org/topics/lgbtq/transgender.pdf

Angelis, C. D., Nardone, A., Garifalos, F., Pivonello, C., Sansone, A., Conforti, A., Dato, C. D., Sirico, F., Alviggi, C., Isidori, A., Colao, A., & Pivonello, R. (2019). Smoke, alcohol and drug addiction and female fertility. *Reproductive Biology and Endocrinology: RB&E, 18*(1), 21. 10.1186/s12958-020-0567-7

Boivin J., Bunting L., Collins J., Nygren K. (2007). International estimates of infertility prevalence and treatment-seeking: potential need and demand for infertility medical care. *Human Reproduction, 22*(6), 1506–1512.

Centers for Disease Control and Prevention. (2021, November 8). *Key statistics from the national survey of family growth – I Listing*. https://www.cdc.gov/nchs/nsfg/key_statistics/i-keystat.htm#infertility

Centers for Disease Control and Prevention. (2022a). *Infertility FAQs*. https://www.cdc.gov/reproductivehealth/infertility/index.htm

Centers for Disease Control and Prevention. (2022b). *STD facts - pelvic inflammatory disease*. https://www.cdc.gov/std/pid/stdfact-pid.htm

Centers for Disease Control and Prevention. (2022c). *Sexually transmitted disease surveillance 2020*. https://www.cdc.gov/std/statistics/2020/default.htm

Centers for Disease Control and Prevention. (2022d). *Women and heart disease*. https://www.cdc.gov/heartdisease/women.htm

Chaer, R., Nakouzi, N., Itani, L., Tannir, H., Kreidieh, D., El Masri, D., & El Ghoch, M. (2020). Fertility and reproduction after recovery from anorexia nervosa: A systematic review and meta-analysis of long-term follow-up studies. *Diseases (Basel, Switzerland)*, *8*(4), 46. 10.3390/diseases8040046

Cleveland Clinic. (2020, December 13). *Infertility causes*. https://my.clevelandclinic.org/health/diseases/16083-infertility-causes

Dağ, Z. Ö., & Dilbaz, B. (2015). Impact of obesity on infertility in women. *Journal of the Turkish German Gynecological Association*, *16*(2), 111–117. 10.5152/jtgga.2015.15232

Doka, K.J. (1989). *Disenfranchised grief: Recognizing hidden sorrow*. Lexington, MA: Lexington Books.

Doka, K. J. (1999). Disenfranchised grief. *Bereavement Care*, *18*(3), 37–39. 10.1080/02682629908657467

Doka, K.J. (2002). *Disenfranchised grief: New challenges, directions, and strategies for practice*. Champaign, IL: Research Press.

Duffy, C., & Allen, S. (2009). Medical and psychosocial aspects of fertility after cancer. *The Cancer Journal*, *15*(1), 27–33. 10.1097/PPO.0b013e3181976602

Hogue, C. J. R. (1986). Impact of abortion on subsequent fecundity. *Clinics in Obstetrics and Gynecology*, *13*(1), 95–103. 10.1016/S0306-3356(21)00156-4

Mughal, S., Azhar, Y., & Siddiqui, W. (2022, July 20). Postpartum depression. In *StatPearls*. StatPearls Publishing. Retrieved October 8, 2022, from https://www.ncbi.nlm.nih.gov/books/NBK519070/

Nillni, Y. I., Wesselink, A. K., Gradus, J. L., Hatch, E. E., Rothman, K. J., Mikkelsen, E. M., & Wise, L. A. (2016). Depression, anxiety, and psychotropic medication use and fecundability. *American Journal of Obstetrics and Gynecology*, *215*(4), 453.e1–453.e4538. 10.1016/j.ajog.2016.04.022

Podfigurna, A., & Meczekalski, B. (2021). Functional hypothalamic amenorrhea: A stress-based disease. *Endocrines*, *2*(3), 203–211. 10.3390/endocrines2030020

Rooney, K. L., & Domar, A. D. (2018). The relationship between stress and infertility. *Dialogues in Clinical Neuroscience*, *20*(1), 41–47. 10.31887/DCNS.2018.20.1/klrooney

Ross J. D. (2013). Pelvic inflammatory disease. *BMJ Clinical Evidence*, *2013*, 1606.

Sarrel, P. M., & DeCherney, A. H. (1985). Psychotherapeutic intervention for treatment of couples with secondary infertility. *Fertility and Sterility*, *43*(6), 897–900. 10.1016/S0015-0282(16)48618-8

Tsevat, D.G., Wiesenfeld, H.C., Parks, C., & Peipert, J.F. (2017). Sexually transmitted diseases and infertility. *American Journal of Obstetrics & Gynecology*, *216*(1):1–9. 10.1016/j.ajog.2016.08.008

Upadhyay, U.D., Johns, N.E., Barron, R., Cartwright, A.F., Tapé, C., Mierjeski, A., & McGregor, A.J. (2018). *BMC Medicine*, *16*(1), 88. 10.1186/s12916-018-1072-0.

U.S. Department of Health and Human Services. (2017). What are some possible causes of female infertility? *Eunice Kennedy Shriver National Institute of Child Health and Human Development*. https://www.nichd.nih.gov/health/topics/infertility/conditioninfo/causes/causes-female

Verit, F. F., Yildiz Zeyrek, F., Zebitay, A. G., & Akyol, H. (2017). Cardiovascular risk may be increased in women with unexplained infertility. *Clinical and Experimental Reproductive Medicine*, *44*(1), 28–32. 10.5653/cerm.2017.44.1.28

Virk, J., Zhang, J., & Olsen, J. (2007). Medical abortion and the risk of subsequent adverse pregnancy outcomes. *New England Journal of Medicine*, *357*(7), 648–653. 10.1056/nejmoa070445

Woodruff T. K. (2008). Making eggs: Is it now or later? *Nature Medicine*, *14*(11), 1190–1191. 10.1038/nm1108-1190

World Health Organization. (2021, November 25). *Abortion*. https://www.who.int/news-room/fact-sheets/detail/abortion

World Health Organization. (2022) *Congenital anomalies*. https://www.who.int/health-topics/congenital-anomalies#tab=tab_1

Zhang, Y., Yan, J., Han, Q., Yang, T., Cai, L., Fu, Y., Cai, X., & Guo, M. (2017). Emergency obstetric hysterectomy for life-threatening postpartum hemorrhage: A 12-year review. *Medicine*, *96*(45), e8443. 10.1097/MD.0000000000008443

CHAPTER SEVEN

Femininity and Social Implications

Who Am I If I'm Not a Mother?

The *Bible* references Sarah, Rachel, and Hannah's barren wombs. Famously, Henry VIII's second wife, Anne Boleyn, lost her life because of her inability to produce a male heir. Although the idea that a woman's value is rooted in her ability to reproduce is archaic, the remnants of this concept – that adulthood must include parenthood – still exist. On a broad scale, countries in which women are not choosing parenthood, such as China, previously governed by single-child or restrictive child policies, now grapple with the unintended consequences, with three to four percent fewer females than males (Fong, 2016). Childless women often face judgment and stigma from those closest to them, adding to the grief associated with infertility and reproductive loss. When women choose to keep fertility struggles private, it leaves them open to assumptions and commentary about why they remain childless. Even remarks by Pope Francis implying that childless couples are selfish illustrate the highly charged societal views on motherhood.

As helping professionals, you, too, are bombarded by messages about motherhood and the value or meaning of this role. Throughout Chapter 7, we will explore the plight of our hero, the childless mother. We will examine the experience of one who craves the role of motherhood, believes in the promise of perpetuating her family, and seeks a child of her own to nurture. This experience is impacted by and seeps into every aspect of her being, including professional, social, and familial contexts, and often most powerfully within the context of her relationship with her partner. Bronfenbrenner (1974) developed a theory in human development, a means of organizing one's external influences and chronological interactions, into a structured model. This model will serve as a guide for exploring the contextual issues a woman, our hero, encounters through her journey of infertility and reproductive loss.

DOI: 10.4324/9781003336402-10

BRONFENBRENNER'S ECOLOGICAL THEORY

Figure 7.1 illustrates Bronfenbrenner's Ecosystem, initially developed to identify factors impacting childhood development, both contextually and chronologically. It is comprised of various systems which impact development based on proximity to the individual. Bronfenbrenner sees the individual as the center point of these contexts. The individual is comprised of multiple personal constructs including sex, age, and health, and is constantly impacted by and impacts their surroundings which are the microsystem, mesosystem, exosystem, macrosystem, and chronosystem. Throughout this chapter, we explore the developmental journey of our hero as an adult and her growth through the journey of infertility and reproductive loss.

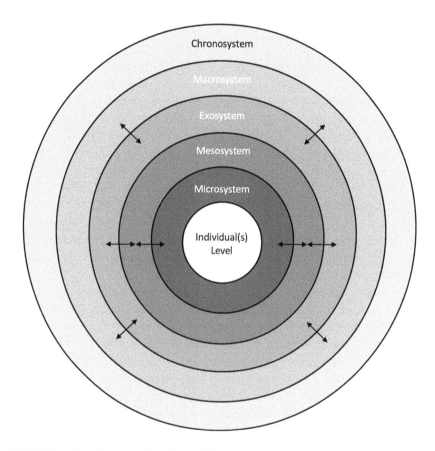

FIGURE 7.1 Bronfenbrenner's Ecological Model

Source: https://commons.wikimedia.org/wiki/File:Bronfenbrenner%27s_Ecological_Model.png

The Individual

The individual, our hero, is at the center of the system, comprised of individual factors inherent to her personality and herself. Often this self was developed in her formative years and may include an inherent desire to be a mother. She may recall herself early in her life, a little girl playing with dolls in preparation for motherhood, with the spontaneous cooing and smiling that comes with seeing a small child. It is this early individual motivation which later results in the crisis of infertility (Taymor & Bresnick, 1979) when not fulfilled. For helping professionals to be successful in providing support and guidance throughout the journey of infertility, it is imperative they are attuned to the idiomatic factors of the individual. The hero's individual self will be further explored through the lens of the RESPECTFUL Model (D'Andrea & Daniels, 1997, 2001) in Chapter 10.

The Microsystem

In the context of Bronfenbrenner's Ecosystem, the microsystem is closest to the individual and has the greatest influence on the hero's experiences. This system consists of the individual's family, friends, professional setting, religious affiliation, and the healthcare system. The interactions between our hero and her microsystem are multi-directional, and for the purpose of this chapter will also include the intimate partner (this construct was not included in Bronfenbrenner's original developmental model, which was used to describe child development).

Intimate Partner

While external experiences amplify the pressure of if and how to successfully conceive following a diagnosis of infertility, the Hero's Journey is likely shared most closely with her intimate partner. A natural, if not optimistic, assumption might be that if two intimate partners are experiencing the same difficulties in achieving parenthood, their experiences would be somewhat similar. However, the experiences of the partner who will be conceiving and bearing the child are often surprisingly distinct from the other prospective parent, not to mention that the methods of medical assistance are drastically different. While both partners in traditional male/female relationships report experiencing sadness and anxiety (Nagórska et al., 2019), the emotional processing is distinct, with women being more likely to attempt to process emotions externally, and men more likely to turn inward. In addition to the individual processing the inability to conceive, acceptance of continuing in a childless marriage tends to be far more acceptable among male partners.

Chapter 10 will focus more directly on marginalized populations, but it is important to reflect upon the barriers for lesbian and gay couples seeking parenthood, as they face additional decision-making challenges than cisgender male and female couples. The emotionally charged decisions related to infertility and reproductive loss, often exacerbated by discrimination and heterosexism, can amplify the emotional distress experienced by these couples. Even within the homosexual community, a hierarchy exists among the beliefs of the general population, with the perception that adoption by a lesbian couple is more acceptable than by two male parents (Patterson, 2005). Partnered with this hierarchy is the ease with which a lesbian couple may conceive compared to a gay couple. One example is the far easier access to donated sperm than eggs (Almeling, 2017). It was not until the 1980s that lesbian couples were regularly accepted by fertility clinics, with increased barriers for their male counterparts regarding access to Assisted Reproductive Technology. Male gay couples often struggle while seeking means of parenthood – generally surrogacy or adoption – and are not immune to emotional difficulties occurring throughout this process in their relationship. As the helping professional guiding heroes and partners through this journey, awareness of the unique experiences of those within the LGBTQ is vital.

RODRIGO'S STORY

Growing up gay you aren't sure if a family of your own is anything more than a dream. Then one day you meet a partner that shares similar values, who is close to their own family, and wants to have kids too. Some dreams do come true.

Soon after we were married in 2018, we attended a seminar for prospective gay families to learn about surrogacy, foster care, and adoption. Surrogacy didn't feel right for us and was probably out of our financial reach. We knew adoption would be the path that we'd pursue.

There are a ton of agencies out there, and not all support gay couples. The agency we chose prided themselves in putting the birth mother first. We felt that aligned with our values. Now that an agency was selected, the real work began including months of gathering personal and financial records. We got our well water tested. We had our house inspected by the fire chief. We got our fingerprints taken for FBI background checks. We prepared an online photo and video profile for prospective families to learn about us. And finally, the dreaded "home visit" which turned out to be a beautiful conversation with our agency rep. Suddenly you're jealous of other couples who don't have to go through all this scrutiny – or wish that some should be required to.

Finally, everything was ready for us to "go live" which means that our online profile was live.

Some people get matched in the first month. Others, after several years. After six months and no matches, it began to feel like a waiting game that would never end. You begin to question your profile, the photos, and videos you chose. In fact, we decided that we needed more videos and enlisted family to help us. Around the holidays, the depression of waiting started to settle in. In January 2020, we began to pray that if there was a soul out there that was looking for a family, we were here waiting, too. Finally, we received a call from our agency that there was a potential match. We learned that we were the only family they were interested in after reading through all of the profiles. They had chosen us! The birth father told us that his best friend was gay, and it was important for his friend to see that he could have his own family one day. We learned she was six months pregnant, and due to their life and family situation, they knew they needed to find a loving family to raise their child.

The time between being matched and the actual birth was its own emotional rollercoaster. This was "our pregnancy". Our birth family was 1,200 miles away, and video calls weren't the norm yet. Because of the birth mother's situation, there were a lot of uncertainties, and our agency probably got tired of our daily emails with never ending questions. Then Covid changed all our lives one month before the due date. During that time, the birth family shared the ultrasound, and we learned that we were having a boy! We decided to take advantage of being able to work remotely and headed to Florida two weeks before his due date in case we needed to quarantine – rules were changing daily.

We met the birth family on Easter Sunday shortly after our arrival. We spent a couple of hours together just getting to know each other. It was a little surreal. Five days later, we received a call early in the morning saying she was in labor. With Covid, we weren't sure if we would be allowed in the hospital as no one besides the birth parents were allowed in. Thankfully, we were allowed in, and we met our son just three hours after he was born. We shared the next three days in the hospital with him just down the hall from the birth parents who we visited with each day.

We were worried about what the hospital experience would be like as a gay adoptive couple. We were told to be sure to bring the nurses cookies – they like cookies. Our hospital went above and beyond and provided us with such amazing service. We still send our nurse a holiday card each year. The moment you see your child for the first time is a moment you never forget. For us, they rolled him into the room shortly after our arrival, said a few things – don't remember what – and left. They left us. Alone. And it was an amazing bonding moment as a family. We instantly became one.

Over the next year we learned to how to be parents during Covid doing all the normal things – but not doing a lot of normal things, too. We've been at it for 2½ years now, and think we are doing pretty good as parents. We have a ton of support from our family. We remain in touch with our birth parents. Each holiday we share photos and videos. We've even received gifts with cards saying how grateful they are for us. We are glad to have this open connection, and only time will tell what that will mean for all of us, including Silas. Adoption is a journey and different for everyone. We've been blessed with ours.

While research provides insight into the emotional experiences of our hero and intimate partner, each couple experiences their own individual journey. If there are no immediate pervasive difficulties, the helping professional can be assured that points of discord will occur. Studies indicate that marital satisfaction may be negatively impacted by an infertility diagnosis (Samadaee-Gelehkolaee et al., 2015). Adjustment to the diagnosis is often depicted by Kubler-Ross's (1969) grieving process, and our hero may experience disenfranchised grief (Doka, 1989, 1999, 2002). Following the diagnosis of infertility, our hero is presented with a bevy of decisions as well as financial and sometimes legal barriers. Like the unique journey of our hero and her partner, the degree to which they share this story with those in their context is varied. Often, private internal struggles occur, while the couple commonly fields questions and comments about when they plan to become parents. This creates an impossible task of managing boundaries and expectations both internally and externally. Few boundaries are more difficult to establish than those between oneself and primary family, or in-laws.

Family

There are few individuals more invested emotionally and biologically in the pregnancy and parenthood of an individual than parents and in-laws. The Harvard Medical School Health Blog refers to parents of those struggling with infertility or pregnancy loss as grandparents in waiting, (Glazer, 2019) and outlines the emotional difficulties and societal pressures associated with this role which may, in turn, impact the relationship with the hero. While often well-intentioned, the direct and implied questions, comments, and interactions with these and other family members may amplify the distress associated with the experience of infertility. In some instances, boundaries between these systems (primary and secondary families) can be blurred while financial and emotional support is offered and at times accepted. These offerings layer the difficulties associated with the hero's infertility with complicated quid pro quo and beholding to outside parties. This can create a unique paradigm in which family members, particularly parents, who may have acted as emotional support in the past, are unable to provide this type of support during the journey of infertility, amplifying the pressures to conceive.

While women may find it simpler to establish boundaries with colleagues, peers, and friends about which events to attend or questions they will field, families can have more complicated relationships. With family, one's pregnancy status is directly related to continuing the bloodline. Often for parents and grandparents of a woman experiencing infertility, there is a personal, even innately driven pressure for a continuation of the lineage. The stakes seem even higher in this context and may become more nuanced and complicated when pressure for children comes from the partner's family. Tension may even be found in sibling relationships, as some continue to have children while their brothers or sisters may not be able to conceive. Parents and grandparents may give more attention to children who have given them grandchildren, leaving those struggling with infertility feeling even more isolated. Coupled with this intense pressure comes the clashing of intergenerational social mores. While 20-something peers might be more attuned to social faux pas associated with direct questioning about having children, those of a different generation, including Baby Boomers or Generation X, may feel less inhibited in expressing their confusion.

Friends

When it comes to social pressure to become a mother, the stakes are raised substantially among friends and acquaintances within the same age group. Research indicates that when individuals start to pair off (or, in our hero's case, some conceive and become parents), others who follow different paths may see these friendships weaken. Lack of shared experience can lead to drifting apart and an increase in isolation and feelings of inadequacy for those facing infertility (Martins et al., 2014; McBain & Reeves, 2019). Essentially, if you aren't having children, and your friends are, these friendships become difficult to sustain. If these friendships *are* sustained, maintaining strong emotional connections with those who are celebrating the milestones associated with becoming pregnant, having children, and celebrating birthdays can be an emotional minefield.

This distancing often places additional pressure on our hero who may feel compelled to support and celebrate friends' pregnancies, while each shower or party is accompanied by internal discomfort and even distress. These events are often arenas for awkward questions from peers regarding future plans to conceive. Following the celebratory experiences associated with becoming pregnant and welcoming a child, the social chasm between those who have children and those who do not often widens. Friendships build on shared experiences, and as friends lose common interests, the all-encompassing role of a parent often defines one friend and not the other. This is a painful reality for our hero as she grapples with the loss of much-needed support systems during her journey of infertility.

Professional Setting

Women of childbearing years may experience professional expectations which exceed those placed on peers who have children such as being asked to stay later or work longer than their colleagues who are parents. Conversely, a woman who chooses not to work and hopes to become pregnant will likely garner her own set of pressures and judgments. Women who prioritized education and careers, placing those pursuits before those of seeking partnership and parenthood during childbearing years, are often placed in a sort of collegial minefield in fielding questions and dealing with assumptions from coworkers.

Although workplace behavior is structured with formal standards for conduct (such as legal ramifications for inquiring about pregnancy status), women struggling with infertility often field subtle and, at times, overt inquiries from professional peers regarding the state of one's potential parenthood. The hero likely struggles with navigating these questions while maintaining professionalism. Despite the primary focus on productivity, the workplace is not devoid of celebrations of milestones among colleagues, including workplace festivities for weddings and baby showers. The blending of these personal and professional boundaries may lead to questions or assumptions about the pregnancy status of a woman grappling with infertility among peers. Also, this extends the avoidable attendance of rituals associated with pregnancy and childbirth in one's social context into unavoidable events within the professional realm.

Religious Affiliation

Despite the recent decline in attendance in traditional churches and synagogues (Jones, 2021), many individuals and families still seek support and a sense of community through participation in attending regular worship ceremonies. Those with whom the hero gathers on a regular basis often grow emotionally bonded to her and with them. It is likely they share a common experience and provide support in times of difficulty and joy and celebration with milestones. Cultural context often exists within the hero's religious affiliation. Are all her peers having children? Is there pressure to conceive? Does she feel compelled to share her fertility journey with this individual, although she may not be comfortable? The helping professional must be attuned to how all these contextual factors related to religious affiliation impact the hero throughout her journey.

Healthcare Services

Following the diagnosis of infertility, our hero finds herself thrust into regular interactions with a bevy of healthcare professionals. As her condition is assessed, diagnosed, and treated, she sees nurses, doctors, and medical technicians through every part of her journey. If she seeks counseling, this group could include you, your student, or the supervisee. Bronfenbrenner includes these individuals as those most intimate and directly impactful to our hero. These providers are human, complete with biases and perceptions about families, babies, and motherhood, all of which can impact our hero.

The Mesosystem

The mesosystem is a combination of two or more components of the microsystem. The interaction between these two may either be of benefit or detriment to our hero. Examples of these include either supportive or critical interactions between those members of the microsystem, for example, the hero's intimate partner and primary family or religious affiliation. According to Bronfenbrenner, positive interactions between these systems act as the catalyst for positive development for a child, and negative interactions impede healthy development. Again, our hero is not a child, but in a place of development in her own right, is impacted similarly by contextual interactions throughout her journey. As helping professionals, we must be cognizant of contextual difficulties in the mesosystem, having awareness of how these negative interactions may be exacerbated by poor boundaries and enmeshment as other members of the mesosystem insert themselves in factors related to the fertility journey (Bowen, 1978).

The Exosystem

The exosystem refers to an environment in which the individual is not directly involved, yet is impacted by its secondary influences. For our hero, this could include pressures experienced by or biases held by members of the microsystem including family, friends, and intimate partner(s) which complicate the interactions between our hero and these members of her microsystem. An example of this is if the hero's intimate partner is having difficulty at their job. This interaction may adversely impact the ability of that partner to support the hero in her infertility journey, amplifying the difficulties of her experience.

The Macrosystem

The macrosystem consists of broad, sometimes abstract societal views and community effects, each of which influences an individual. While the somewhat abstract nature of the macrosystem may seem irrelevant to our hero, Bronfenbrenner would indicate otherwise. The macrosystem impacts beliefs and behaviors on a large scale for our hero and those in her periphery. These constructs of the macrosystem are dynamic, changing with time and societal political trends. Examples of these include views on women's rights, the definition of a family, and community effects. We can see clear delineations in our macrosystem of 2022 and that of the macrosystem of 100 years ago. Previously, women were sequestered to their roles as wives and mothers, rarely working outside the home, and only recently allowed to vote. Widely held political views on race, gender, and equality all fall into this category and are likely to influence our hero and her interactions with her more proximate systems. In Chapter 10 we will look more closely at how varying intersections of our hero's characteristics and her macrosystem interact.

Societal Views

The childless mother … this term alone is an oxymoron. How does society view the individual who, like our hero, struggles with this concept? Can she be a mother without the presence of a child to nurture? Is motherhood something we do, or is it who we are? Without tapping too deeply into the philosophy of post-constructivist definitions, understanding this role, how it is developed, and how it is viewed provides insight into how our hero is impacted by societal views through her fertility journey. Research associated with understanding the individual desire for parenthood identifies universal factors, consistent across genders, sexual identities, and those who chose not to have children. Often, the meaning of making one's life is tied directly to the choice to have children, both for those who seek to procreate, and those who intentionally avoid parenthood (Khazan, 2021). We would be remiss in failing to recognize how the drive to strive for and meet societal standards and expectations shapes this decision.

Community Effects

A recent study (van Balen & Bos, 2009) described community effect factors associated with infertility including loss of status, ridicule, stigmatization, isolation, and rejection. These effects occurred on a spectrum from low-level to intense experiences but were rarely absent altogether. Within the context of her community, the childless mother is often devoid of the respect and recognition shown to her peers with children – resulting in a negative sense of self, isolation, and estrangement from the community. This provides a basis for understanding the broad cultural experiences of our hero experiencing infertility, that even if minimal, they are nearly omnipotent among women who are not mothers. Implicit messages from religious organizations, politicians, and even social media often extol the values of parenthood and the value of those who have children, conversely marginalizing those who do not (Öztürk et al., 2021). You, the helping professionals guiding the hero through her journey, may consider the possible benefits of psychoeducation related to these large-scale issues. Exploring these community influences with our hero may help with meaning-making about messages she receives related to her infertility journey.

The Chronosystem

Finally, Bronfenbrenner's chronosystem integrates the passage of time into the developmental model, delineating between two major chronological components, normative and nonnormative life transitions. The divide between these two strikes at the heart of this book. Normative life transitions are the fulfillment and completion of a variety of milestones in a predictable manner. These nearly always happen. Individuals regularly graduate from school, move out of their parents' homes, get a job, find a partner, and start a family. Our hero has likely progressed through many normative components, milestones associated with growing from childhood to adulthood. At the point that she determined that she wanted to become a mother and was unable to do so, she began to experience nonnormative life transitions, disrupting the expected progression. It is these nonnormative experiences that deviate from the general experience, isolating our hero from the norm. It is often at this time that our hero begins to grieve the loss of these normative models and begins to experience disenfranchised grief (Doka, 1989, 1999, 2002) associated with this loss.

Why are we motivated to have children? The answer to this question is multifaceted and provides clarity on why those having trouble conceiving are motivated to traverse a multitude of physical, emotional, and financial hurdles to achieve the desired outcome of parenthood. This innate desire, independent of societal and familial pressures, can be broken down into two primary categories. One part of the motivation to be a mother is rational and easily verbalized, while the other motivation may originate more from an intrinsic desire which is less easily articulated but more profound. When asked to describe this need, one might logically outline the need to fulfill the American dream, create a legacy, expand one's family, or ensure they are cared for as they age. More existential motivations may be less easily verbalized but might include finding or making meaning in one's life, replicating a happy childhood, or breaking the cycle of unhappiness experienced in their childhood.

CONCLUSION

Chapter 7 explored those factors which influence our hero through her journey to motherhood. Motherhood, and all that it carries, is synergistic. Our hero, seeking the role of mother, may experience individual, intimate partner, family, and societal challenges when grappling with infertility. Bronfenbrenner's Ecosystem provides structure to the contextual issues impacting our hero through her journey of infertility. Her very personal experiences are not impervious to external effects. Our hero's world is not only contextual, but chronological, including influences from the microsystem, mesosystem, exosystem, macrosystem, and chronosystem. Understanding the many contexts of the hero and bringing these constructs to her attention can aid you as you guide her through her journey of infertility and reproductive loss.

REFERENCES

Almeling, R. (2017). The business of egg and sperm donation. *Contexts*, *16*(4), 68–70. 10.1177/1536504217742396

Bowen, M. (1978) *Family therapy in clinical practice*. New York: Jason Aronson, Inc.

Bronfenbrenner, U. (1974). Developmental research, public policy, and the ecology of childhood. *Child Development*, *45*(1), 1–5. 10.2307/1127743

D'Andrea, M., & Daniels, J. (1997). Multicultural counseling supervision: Central issues, theoretical considerations, and practical strategies. In D.B. Pope-Davis & H.L.K. Coleman (Eds.), *Multicultural Competencies: Assessment, Education and Training, and Supervision* (pp. 290–309). Thousand Oaks, CA: Sage.

D'Andrea, M., & Daniels, J. (2001). Respectful counseling: An integrative multidimensional model for counselors. In D. Pope-Davis, & H. Coleman (Eds.), *The Intersection of Race, Class, and Gender in Multicultural Counseling* (pp. 417–466). SAGE Publications, Inc., 10.4135/9781452231846.n17

Doka, K.J. (1989). *Disenfranchised grief: Recognizing and treating hidden sorrow*. Jossey-Bass Publishers.

Doka, K.J. (1999). Disenfranchised grief. *Bereavement Care*, *18*(3), 37–39. 10.1080/02682629908657467

Doka, K.J. (2002). *Disenfranchised grief: New challenges, directions, and strategies for practice*. Champaign, IL: Research Press.

Fong, M. (2016). *One child: The story of China's most radical experiment*. Houghton Mifflin Harcourt Publishing Company.

Glazer, E.S. (2019, December 17). *Infertility: Grandparents in waiting*. Harvard Health. https://www.health.harvard.edu/blog/infertility-grandparents-in-waiting-2019121718540

Jones, J.M. (2021, November 20). *U.S. church membership falls below majority for first time*. Gallup. https://news.gallup.com/poll/341963/church-membership-falls-below-majority-first-time.aspx

Khazan, O. (2021, May 25). *How people decide whether to have children*. The Atlantic. https://www.theatlantic.com/health/archive/2017/05/how-people-decide-whether-to-have-children/527520/

Kubler-Ross, E. (1969). *On death and dying*. Scribner.

Martins, M.V., Costa, P., Peterson, B.D., Costa, M.E., & Schmidt, L. (2014). Marital stability and repartnering: Infertility-related stress trajectories of unsuccessful fertility treatment. *Fertility and Sterility*, *102*(6), 1716–1722. 10.1016/j.fertnstert.2014.09.007

McBain, T.D., & Reeves, P. (2019). Women's experience of infertility and disenfranchised grief. *The Family Journal*, *27*(2), 156–166. 10.1177/1066480719833418

Nagórska, M., Bartosiewicz, A., Obrzut, B., & Darmochwał-Kolarz, D. (2019). Gender differences in the experience of infertility concerning Polish couples: Preliminary research. *International Journal of Environmental Research and Public Health*, *16*(13), 2337. 10.3390/ijerph16132337

Öztürk, R., Bloom, T.L., Li, Y., & Bullock, L.F.C. (2021). Stress, stigma, violence experiences and social support of US infertile women. *Journal of Reproductive & Infant Psychology*, *39*(2), 205–217. 10.1080/02646838.2020.1754373

Patterson, C. (2005). *Lesbian and gay parenting: Theoretical and conceptual examinations*. American Psychological Association. https://www.apa.org/pi/lgbt/resources/parenting

Samadaee-Gelehkolaee, K., McCarthy, B.W., Khalilian, A., Hamzehgardeshi, Z., Peyvandi, S., Elyasi, F., & Shahidi, M. (2015). Factors associated with marital satisfaction in infertile couple: A comprehensive literature review. *Global Journal of Health Science*, *8*(5), 96–109. 10.5539/gjhs.v8n5p96

Taymor, M.L., & Bresnick, E. (1979). Emotional stress and infertility. *Infertility*, *2*(1), 39–47.

van Balen, F., & Bos, H.M. (2009). The social and cultural consequences of being childless in poor-resource areas. *Facts, Views & Vision in ObGyn*, *1*(2), 106–121.

CHAPTER EIGHT

Male Factor Infertility

Dude, Am I Shooting Blanks?

What if our hero is a guy?

Throughout this book, the focus has been placed on the female hero and her infertility journey. This well-deserved place at the forefront of our focus is rooted in biology and societal roles. In this chapter, we shift focus to the male's journey of infertility and reproductive loss. What are his experiences associated with biological limitations to conceiving? What are his experiences in an intimate relationship with a partner who cannot conceive? Similar to the link between femininity and motherhood, male infertility may adversely impact self-worth, even masculinity. While a man's ability to reproduce is not as directly correlated to aging as a woman's, other factors such as heredity, disease, and injury may play a role. Research suggests that men are less likely to conflate masculinity and gender identity with an inability to reproduce than their female counterparts. However, the diagnosis of infertility still brings psychological and relational ramifications. Similar to female infertility, a male partner may experience infertility quite differently, exacerbating his struggle. In this chapter, we explore a variety of aspects related to the experience of male infertility.

MALE INFERTILITY

Men are parents, too, half of the equation. The desire to procreate, long associated with women, is now becoming recognized as a shared experience between partners, men and women alike. Motivators such as the fulfillment of becoming a parent, continuing one's bloodline, and creating a family are values not attributable to one sex (Langdridge et al., 2005). The brunt of the responsibility of conception through pregnancy and birth (and sometimes beyond), falls

DOI: 10.4324/9781003336402-11

on the biological mother, and therefore societal focus follows. Somewhat universally, social mores define and celebrate women by their role as mothers and caretakers.

This tendency to focus on only one parent (the mother) is likely the result of small- and large-scale contextual issues, as discussed in Chapter 7. These factors are evident in the primarily female-centric cultural rituals such as baby showers and sprinkles and legal structures like the Family Medical Leave Act which have historically focused on maternity leave. Things are changing, and societal inclusion of the man is transitioning from the Norman Rockwell depiction of a proud father handing out cigars in the hospital waiting room after the delivery of his child. Modern celebrations and recognition of the value of the father are becoming more common, including couples' showers and the advent of the progression of paternity leave. Trends of inclusiveness, more equal parenting, and a shared desire for parenthood require the helping professional's recognition of these changes and aptitude to counsel males seeking parenthood.

What if it's his plumbing? Societal standards aside, the presence of a male's physical contribution to conception is a biological necessity and one that is becoming an increasingly relevant component in infertility research. In recent years, there has been a substantial focus on male infertility (Baskaran et al., 2021). Like the potential physical limitations in conception for women, male infertility plays a role in between one-third (Fronczak et al., 2012) and one-half of fertility issues (Agarwal et al., 2015). When a couple comes to realize the presence of fertility problems, often the initial focus is on the female. Initial diagnosis occurs when pregnancy is not achieved within one year of unprotected intercourse or one year of therapeutic donor insemination (The American College of Obstetricians and Gynecologists, 2019). Despite the substantial portion of infertility associated with males, this population is often initially overlooked.

Following the exploration and elimination of the female's role in the diagnosis of infertility, the possibility of male-factor infertility is explored. It is at this point that our male hero starts to ponder his role, perhaps his masculinity, desire for fatherhood, and the likelihood he will become a parent. Male infertility diagnoses may be attributed to a variety of factors including congenital issues, injuries such as testicular trauma, cancer and associated treatments, diabetes, cystic fibrosis, and auto-immune disorders. Hormonal issues and genetic disorders also impact male sperm count and subsequent ability to conceive (Elfateh et al., 2014). In some instances, a man has determined he has finished having children and taken steps to prevent conception such as vasectomy, and has to seek a reversal. Finally, although not as directly correlated to fertility issues as female aging, paternal age does play a role in sperm production and the ability to conceive.

While several of the male factor infertility components are genetic, many are attributed to lifestyle choices and, therefore, potentially resolved through behavior modification. Recreational drug use, tobacco, caffeine, and alcohol use, as well as obesity and the onset of type 2 diabetes, have adverse effects on fertility. Specifically, weekly marijuana use in males has been linked to lower sperm count and an increase in erectile dysfunction (Srinivasan et al., 2021). Again, this information may be relevant for you as the helping professional and our male hero as he begins his journey through infertility and reproductive loss. Our hero may benefit from behavioral modification interventions such as smoking cessation and the development of alternative coping skills within the context of therapy to increase the likelihood of conception.

Similar to the perspective we took in Chapter 7 regarding how a woman's infertility journey is impacted greatly by those in her periphery, we must also explore the male partner and her experience as her partner struggles with a diagnosis. Does she serve as a support to him? Do blame and resentment occur? How is this impacting their relationship? This chapter is unique in its focus on our hero as a male, not only as a part of a couple grappling with infertility but as an individual as well.

Age-Related Male Infertility

Although age-related infertility is typically attributed to women, it does play a role in the conception of children for males later in life (Harris et al., 2011). This diagnosis is complicated and includes a number of factors integral to our understanding of the male hero. Aging brings a variety of issues to the table. Men who are aging typically have aging partners, they have had more opportunity for exposure to environmental factors leading to infertility, and they have lower libido, all of which can create difficulties with fertility. The helping professional's attunement to intimate partner and family systems perspectives is imperative here, as well as awareness of how aging and age-related infertility can be the catalyst for an existential crisis for our male hero.

Although in rare instances men are able to father children into their 70s and even 80s, the concept that men can father children at any age is a myth, perhaps one that our hero bought into. Not only is male infertility a factor in between one-third and half of couples with infertility, but since the 1980s, trends in male infertility have increased significantly (Kumar & Singh, 2015). As helping professionals, it is important to remember that our hero can be impacted by age-related infertility and understand the emotional ramifications for both he and his partner.

Non-Age-Related Male Infertility

Men, even young men, are struggling with infertility. In the medical community, non-age-related male fertility can fall into three different categories. These are congenital, acquired, and idiopathic. While it may be unnecessary for helping professionals to delve too deeply into the physiological components related to non-age-related male infertility, it is imperative that we are aware of these issues in order to effectively support clients. Chromosomal abnormalities and genetic malformations associated with diseases such as cystic fibrosis and Kallmann Syndrome which limit sperm production are examples of some congenital factors related to infertility (Agarwal et al., 2021). Acquired fertility factors related to environment or lifestyle such as those mentioned earlier in the chapter (tobacco use, alcohol use, obesity, and injury) also fall under this umbrella as well as cancers and other non-congenital diseases. Finally, in some instances, idiopathic factors involve finding no identifiable factors for the male or his partner, leaving our hero at an emotional loss with no explanation about the cause.

EMOTIONAL CONSEQUENCES OF MALE INFERTILITY

Boys don't cry. This sentence is both a lyric (The Cure, 1980) and a nod to antiquated views on the male expression of emotion. While the earlier part of this chapter focused on the medical factors associated with male factor infertility, the remainder will focus on the way in which males dealing with infertility experience their journey individually and as part of an intimate partnership. Emotional, psychological, social, and financial consequences associated with infertility are not limited to female heroes. In some instances, the issue is not a male or female problem but one that the couple shares as an entity. While it is imperative that helping professionals remain open to how the issue of infertility impacts all parties involved, we must maintain awareness of how the person who holds responsibility for the infertility diagnosis may be impacted. If the diagnostic intervention identifies a "faulty" party, the emotional ramifications of the diagnosis can be amplified.

There is no doubt that infertility is an emotionally charged experience for men (Sherrod, 2006), often resulting in depression and anxiety (Yang et al., 2017). Distinct from the garnering of support and external processing of their female partners, men have a tendency to turn inward during this journey. Frequently, as a result of concealing and internalizing emotions, men handle emotional crises through culturally sanctioned activities in line with the damaging concept that men don't cry. The expression of negative emotions in males remains somewhat socially unacceptable, viewed as weak or feminine. More acceptable means of expression include anger and frustration than grief and sadness (National Institute of Mental Health, 2017). This male emotional experience is so distinct that in 1995, Sherrod coined the term *the disguise* for his behavior when grappling with infertility.

The disguise encompasses three specific ways in which men respond when faced with infertility. The three ways include disguise to protect self, disguise to protect partner, and disguise to protect both self and partner (Sherrod, 1995). A male grappling with an infertility diagnosis might downplay his desire to have children to focus on work or social aspects, indicating that those distractions make him forget about the issue. He may minimize his emotions within the context of his partner, projecting strength and stoicism, so he won't upset her further. To protect himself and his partner, he may inflate the strength of the relationship, indicating that they are unique, impervious to the emotional impact of infertility. The primary goal of using the disguise in response to infertility is to avoid the emotional turmoil associated with the diagnosis. This self-preservation technique disguises males' feelings from themselves, their partners, and families and most importantly, health care professionals. Awareness of this tendency to disguise is imperative to the work of the helping professional.

TIMOTHY'S STORY

I had always thought I was a healthy guy, played sports in high school, and even intramural sports in college. I could stay up late and still get up and make my day happen. Work hard, play hard. In 2007, I was 24 years old, had my first job, and felt like I was on top of the world. I was living my best life and had a job in my field of study. I wasn't in a serious relationship but was doing my fair share of dating. I started to notice some physical symptoms and honestly ignored them for some time. I had some swelling and heaviness but thought it would just go away. After talking to my brother, he convinced me to go see someone, and in 2008 I was diagnosed with testicular cancer. It was Stage 1 at that point. I was shocked to know that I could have a diagnosis of cancer so early and even more shocked that I would have to undergo treatment. Since it was caught relatively early, interventions were minimal, and the prognosis for survival was good. At that point, having children or a family wasn't on my mind at all. I knew from the doctors that I could have trouble having kids in the future, but I was more focused on survival. I met my wife in 2010, and we married. I was forthcoming with her about my cancer diagnosis. We ended up using a sperm donor and her egg, and our son Anthony was born in 2014. I rarely think of him as different but do feel some jealousy as my wife is able to share his DNA and I am not. It has been a difficult journey for the three of us. But we are a family and that is what matters.

MALE RELATIONSHIPS

Compared to the bevy of research available related to the emotional and social ramifications of female infertility, a true scarcity exists related to the emotional and interpersonal experiences of males suffering from the condition. Most of the empirical research focuses on female infertility with a secondary focus on the impact on males or males as a part of a couple experiencing infertility. The limited research speaks to how often infertility is recognized as a universal female problem. However, recently this trend has been shifting. Academically and culturally, we are starting to place more focus on male infertility and its ramifications (Baskaran et al., 2021). Awareness of the diagnosis is growing along with its multi-faceted impacts on intimate and familial relationships.

Intimate Partner Relationships

Male factor infertility brings about a complicated set of factors for the helping professional to consider. Hanna and Gough (2017) found that men felt a lower degree of agency and sought out less support when dealing with infertility. This could be associated with feelings of emasculation and shame associated with the diagnosis of a traditionally female problem. These feelings, as well as the contextual stigma associated with male infertility such as "shooting blanks" may cause men to isolate. Earlier in the chapter, we mentioned Sherrod's term *the disguise* which refers to the male tendency to hide or disguise his true response to the diagnosis of infertility. As the helping professional, the presence of this phenomenon reiterates the need to explore the way in which each partner experiences the journey of infertility, with attention to how different male and female experiences can be. Research indicates that men report their partners had more of a *need* to have a child than they did and that they felt as if they were unable to support their partner through this journey as the masculine rock of the family. This supportive role can be a source of additional stress when faced with the inability to solve or fix the infertility diagnosis (Taebi et al., 2021).

Research indicates that the way in which a diagnosis of infertility is processed among men and women is inherently distinct. Men tend to process the issue internally and women externally by talking to their partners. This distinction exacerbates the individual stress of diagnosis, resulting in interrelational stress (Gibson & Myers, 2000). The female "unloading", or engaging in external processing of emotional experience, is often a source of increased anxiety for males with an infertility diagnosis (Gibson & Myers, 2000). The helping professional is charged with the heavy task of integrating the internal experiences of the male suffering from infertility and the impact of his partner's experience, as well as discrepancies in their shared experience.

A tendency exists to generalize female and male proclivities, both of which are characterized in the bestselling book, *Men are from Mars, Women are from Venus* (Gray, 1992). Traditionally, women are characterized as seeking physical and emotional support when faced with a problem, and men are charged with coming to the rescue, leaving both sides feeling slighted. Although some tenets of these traditional male and female constructs seem somewhat antiquated, many men and women still struggle with the distinct manner in which they process issues. An acute point in the journey for our hero and his partner is often when avenues to fertility are blocked or when procedures fail. It is at this point that the helping professional must be particularly attuned to how different sexes respond to this situation, the emergence of the disguise in our male hero, and feelings of isolation in his partner.

Family Relationships

In Chapter 6, we focused on the contextual issues of women suffering from infertility. Women, particularly in less Westernized cultures, are more likely to experience severe consequences from parents and partners' parents with the diagnosis of infertility. The degree to which this can occur is illustrated in the title of the article *"My Mother-in-law Forced My Husband to Divorce Me"*: *Experiences of Women with Infertility in Zamfara State of Nigeria* (Naab et al., 2019). A woman's infertility was cause enough for the dissolution of marriage in this 2019 study. Despite the profound impact infertility can have on female identity and contextual interactions, little data exists related to the pressures and judgments placed on males struggling with infertility by primary family, extended family, coworkers, or socially. Perhaps this is attributed to the familial value placed on motherhood or to the unique way in which males disguise their experiences (Sherrod, 1995). However, the lack of data does not indicate men are impervious to these factors.

CONCLUSION

Between one-third and one-half of conception issues can be attributed to male factor infertility. Throughout this chapter, we explored the origins of this type of infertility including congenital, acquired, and idiopathic causes. We also described the experiences of the often-forgotten male partner in a couple struggling with infertility. We focused on biological factors contributing to male factor infertility, difficulties associated with males as a part of a couple with an infertility diagnosis, and the inherent difficulties of the homosexual male. The experiences of males suffering from infertility are distinct from their female counterparts, and a tendency to hide or internalize emotions for our male hero may create an internal, intimate partner, and familial distress during his difficult journey. He requires unique evidence-based intervention from the helping professional to aid him as he travels this path.

REFERENCES

Agarwal, A., Baskaran, S., Parekh, N., Chak-Lam, C., Henkel, R., Vij, S., Arafa, M., Manesh Kumar, P.S., & Shah, R. (2021). Male infertility. *The Lancet*, *397*(10271), 319–333. 10.1016/S0140-6736(20)32667-2

Agarwal, A., Mulgund, A., Hamada, A., & Chyatte, M.R. (2015). A unique view on male infertility around the globe. *Reproductive Biology and Endocrinology: RB&E*, *13*, 37. 10.1186/s12958-015-0032-1

Baskaran, S., Agarwal, A., Leisegang, K., Pushparaj, P.N., Panner Selvam, M.K., & Henkel, R.(2021). An in-depth bibliometric analysis and current perspective on male infertility research. *The World Journal of Men's Health*, *39*(2), 302–314. 10.5534/wjmh.180114

Elfateh, F., Wang, R., Zhang, Z., Jiang, Y., Chen, S., & Liu, R. (2014). Influence of genetic abnormalities on semen quality and male fertility: A four-year prospective study. *Iranian Journal of Reproductive Medicine*, *12*(2), 95–102. https://www.ncbi.nlm.nih.gov/pmc/articles/PMC4009560/

Fronczak, C.M., Kim, E.D., & Barqawi, A.B. (2012). The insults of illicit drug use on male fertility. *Journal of Andrology*, *33*(4), 515–528. 10.2164/jandrol.110. 011874

Gibson, D.M., & Myers, J.E. (2000). Gender and infertility: A relational approach to counseling women. *Journal of Counseling & Development*, *78*(4), 400–410. 10.1002/j.1556-6676.2000.tb01923.x

Gray, J. (1992). *Men are from Mars, women are from Venus: A practical guide for improving communication and getting what you want in your relationships*. HarperCollins.

Hanna, E., & Gough, B. (2017). Men's accounts of infertility within their intimate partner relationships: An analysis of online forum discussions. *Journal of Reproductive and Infant Psychology*, *35*(2), 150–158. 10.1080/02646838. 2017.1278749

Harris, I.D., Fronczak, C., Roth, L., & Meacham, R.B. (2011). Fertility and the aging male. *Reviews in Urology*, *13*(4), 184–190.

Kumar, N., & Singh, A.K. (2015). Trends of male factor infertility, an important cause of infertility: A review of literature. *Journal of Human Reproductive Sciences*, *8*(4), 191–196. 10.4103/0974-1208.170370

Langdridge, D., Sheeran, P., & Connolly, K. (2005). Understanding the reasons for parenthood. *Journal of Reproductive and Infant Psychology*, *23*(2), 121–133. 10.1080/02646830500129438

Naab, F., Lawali, Y., & Donkor, E.S. (2019). "My mother in-law forced my husband to divorce me": Experiences of women with infertility in Zamfara State of Nigeria. *PLoS ONE*, *14*(12). 10.1371/journal.pone.0225149

National Institute of Mental Health. (2017). *Men and Depression*. U.S. Department of Health and Human Services. https://www.nimh.nih.gov/health/publications/men-and-depression

Sherrod, R.A. (1995). A male perspective on infertility. *MCN: The American Journal of Maternal Child Nursing*, *20*(5), 269–275.

Sherrod, R.A. (2006). Male infertility: The element of disguise. *Journal of Psychosocial Nursing and Mental Health Services*, *44*(10), 30–37. 10.3928/02793695-20061001-05

Srinivasan, M., Hamouda, R.K., Ambedkar, B., Arzoun, H.I., Sahib, I., Fondeur, J., Mendez, L.E., & Mohammed, L. (2021) The effect of marijuana on the incidence and evolution of male infertility: A systematic review. *Cureus 13*(12): e20119. 10.7759/cureus.20119

Taebi, M., Kariman, N., Montazeri, A., & Alavi Majd, H. (2021). Infertility stigma: A qualitative study on feelings and experiences of infertile women. *International Journal of Fertility & Sterility*, *15*(3), 189–196. 10.22074/IJFS.2021.139093.1039

The American College of Obstetricians and Gynecologists (2019, May 23). *Infertility workup for the women's health specialist*. https://www.acog.org/clinical/clinical-guidance/committee-opinion/articles/2019/06/infertility-workup-for-the-womens-health-specialist

The Cure. (1980). Boys Don't Cry [Song]. *On Three Imaginary Boys*. [Album]. Fiction: London.

Yang, B., Zhang, J., Yuxia, Q., Wang, P., Ronghuan, J., & Li, H. (2017). Assessment on occurrences of depression and anxiety and associated risk factors in the infertile Chinese men. *American Journal of Men's Health*, *11*(3), 767–774. 10.1177/1557988

CHAPTER NINE

Personal Choices in Growing a Nontraditional Family

Will You Stop Asking Me About Children?

The growth of the American population is at its lowest rate for the first time since the formation of the country (Rogers, 2021). In this chapter, we discuss reasons for that trend, including the fact that many people are intentionally choosing not to have children. Despite an increasing number of those who are choosing to remain childless, a common assumption still exists that almost everyone, particularly those in committed partnerships, will have kids. These assumptions are often made without considering that the person may not want children … or, in the case of our hero, that they desperately want them but can't. In this chapter, we'll explore social pressures for motherhood, the changing American family, nontraditional routes to parenthood, and how the hero can respond when asked about having children.

SOCIAL PRESSURES FOR MOTHERHOOD

Society is changing the way it views traditional gender roles. While these changes have ushered in varying attitudes about parenthood, men and women still experience social pressures when they deviate from the primary role of mother or father (Orth, 2022). These pressures originate from several sources including pronatalist policies, media, and friends and family.

Pronatalist Policies

Pronatalists are defined as people or groups of people who encourage increased birth rates (Merriam-Webster, n.d.). Pronatalist practices are often found in governments that encourage childbearing to support higher birth rates

DOI: 10.4324/9781003336402-12

in their countries. Shechter (2019) posits that pronatalism promotes childbearing for a nation's political, economic, and social purposes and outlines more than a century of public campaigns to persuade women in America to have children. These include Roosevelt's push for Americans to bear children during immigration surges in the early 1900s and the coining of the term biological clock in the 1970s in response to threats of declining fertility when birth rates dropped due to increased usage of birth control. More recently, others explored ways in which decreasing fertility and an increasing elderly population will impact economics and the standard of living, such as the possibility of not having enough people to man the future workforce and support an aging population (Lee & Mason, 2014). Therefore, the push for childbearing may continue. And just in case you were wondering, the United States is not the only country that has embraced pronatalism. In recent years, pro-birth policies have been on the rise in countries such as Latvia, Hungary, Greece, Poland, Japan, Korea, and Finland (Stone, 2020).

While some nations encourage childbearing, pressure to establish a family is often amplified by membership in organized religion. For example, Mormon theology is centered around the idea of eternal families and encourages conception among its followers (Heaton, 1998). Other pronatalist religions include Catholicism and Judaism whose doctrines teach that children are created in the divine image of God and are a blessing from God. It's interesting to note statistics related to birth rates for various religions. Mormons have the highest birth rate (3.4 children), followed by Black Protestants (2.5 children), Evangelical Protestants (2.3 children), Catholics (2.3 children), Jews (2.0), and mainline Protestants (1.9 children) (Ingraham, 2015). It may be beneficial for helping professionals to explore religious affiliation, if any, and how this may impact the pressure our hero feels to have children.

Media

Media also adds pressure to propagate. Books, television, movies, magazines, music, and social media lead many individuals to believe that parenthood is an expected part of the life course. Let's examine a few examples from television, music, and social media.

First, consider television and music. Over the last few decades, television shows such as *Leave It to Beaver*, *The Brady Bunch*, *Family Matters*, *Modern Family*, and *This is Us* depicted family life as the norm. And when it comes to music, you probably hum along to song after song on your playlist about the parenting experience including *Isn't She Lovely*, *In My Daughter's Eyes*, *You're Going to Miss This*, *Blue*, and *Sweetest Devotion*. While many of you reading this book probably weren't even born yet, when it comes to music, we, children of the 80s, can't forget Atlantic Starr's number one hit *Always* which contained lyrics about the unfailing joys of creating and being a part of a family (Atlantic Starr, 1987).

In addition to television and music, social media plays a major role in shaping ideas of who we are and what we are told we should be. According to a 2021 Pew Research report, at least 72% of adults currently use social media, with numbers projected to rise. Many of these adults engage in sharenting, a colloquial term used to describe the habitual sharing of information about one's children through social media. All it takes are a few scrolls through popular social media sites to see post after post of pregnancy announcements, ultrasound photos, gender reveals, baby showers, birth announcements, and milestones such as first steps, first days of school, and graduations. These posts can contribute to added pressure, making it seem as if parenting is the norm. Even in a society where many individuals and couples are choosing to remain childless, social media could lead them to feel they are missing the boat.

Friends and Family

We can't end the discussion about pressures for parenthood without mentioning friends and family. Research conducted on the social demographics of fertility indicated that contact with family, friends, and acquaintances swayed decisions about parenthood including when couples become parents, ideal family size, and the acceptability of adoption and remaining childless (Bernardi & Klarner, 2014). Social pressure may come directly from family members in the form of questions such as, "When are you going to make me a grandparent?", or "When are you going to give Jonah a cousin?" Pressure may also come more subtly. Individuals may see their friends getting married and having children and feel left out of the mix. Maybe they see their parents aging and feel guilty about not giving them the opportunity to have grandchildren. Maybe they wonder who will take care of them when they are old. Whatever the case, it seems that women feel this pressure more than men. Results of one poll indicated that 40% of American women felt pressure to have children, while only 10% of men did (Orth, 2022). Despite a changing society regarding its views of the roles of women and motherhood, it seems most women haven't fully embraced the message.

Pronatalism, media, and friends and family can contribute to pressures for parenthood. Some people succumb to these pressures. And some people truly do want to become parents on their own accord. For those who do, they may experience additional dissonance when their desires conflict with changing societal attitudes regarding having children. In the next section, we discuss these changing societal attitudes and the current landscape of the changing American family.

THE CHANGING AMERICAN FAMILY

The makeup of the typical American family is shifting. In 2021, the U.S. population grew by only 0.1% which is the slowest rate of growth in its history (Rogers, 2021). International migration, increasing mortality rates due to aging, the COVID-19 pandemic, and the decreasing birth rate are the main contributors to this growing trend.

For the past eight years, birth rates and fertility rates have been steadily declining (Hoffower, 2022). One reason might be increased access to birth control, but other factors include simply choosing childlessness. Reasons for this choice include the continued empowerment of women who have the freedom to pursue other paths to fulfillment, rising costs of having a family, postponement of having children, and a growing number of people who say they just don't want children (Hoffower, 2022). Because of these factors, it's no surprise that we see fewer men and women becoming parents. Let's start with access to birth control.

Birth Control

Birth control pills were developed in the 1950s, and since that time, their use has become more widespread. In 2019, 49% of women around the world ranging in age from 15 to 49 years (a total of 922 million women) were using some form of contraception. This is an increase from 42% (a total of 554 million women) in 1990 (United Nations Department of Economics and Social Affairs, 2020). At the same time, statistics indicate that countries with more women using contraception have lower fertility rates (United Nations Department of Economics and Social Affairs, 2020), creating an inverse correlation between the two. For example, in 1990, there were 3.2 live births per woman globally, and in 2019, there were 2.5. This rate is predicted to reach 2.2 per woman in 2050 and 1.9 per woman in 2100 (United Nations Department of Economics and Social Affairs, 2020). Some find this a cause for concern because close to half of all people around the world live in an area where lifetime fertility is below 2.1 live births per woman, which is roughly the level required for populations with low mortality to have a growth rate of zero in the long run (United Nations Department of Economics and Social Affairs, 2020). However, many women continue to use contraception to either limit or prevent children, and this trend will more than likely continue.

Choosing Childlessness

Another reason birth rates are declining is that many individuals are choosing not to have children. In the past, there was a cultural expectation that women would become wives and mothers. Today, these roles are not assumed (Bolick, 2016; Daum, 2015). Many women feel empowered to pursue their careers, travel, hobbies, and other activities they enjoy, and that brings a sense of satisfaction and fulfillment outside of traditional roles. They also tend to feel less stigma from others regarding these choices than their counterparts did in the past. Other reasons for choosing childlessness include the rising costs associated with raising a family, the uncertainty of the world, environmental reasons such as climate change, seeing their lives as complete without children, and just not wanting children. Of non-parents between the ages of 18 to 49, 44% say it's not too likely or not at all likely that children will be part of their future (Brown, 2021). When asked why, 17% cited financial reasons, 9% cited the state of the world, and 5% cited environmental reasons. Additionally, 56% of non-parents below the age of 50 who say it's unlikely they will have kids say they just don't want them (Brown, 2021).

Increased use of birth control and a growing number of people choosing childlessness have led to decreases in the birth rate. However, while many individuals are choosing not to become parents, there remains a large population of those who want to have children … but can't. In the next section, we'll explore some nontraditional routes to parenthood that can assist these individuals with building their families.

NONTRADITIONAL ROUTES TO PARENTHOOD

Alternative routes to parenthood further complicate internal and social pressures about how or if we become parents … or if it is the right decision. In this section, we explore personal choices and nontraditional options regarding parenthood. These include fertility treatments, egg and sperm donation, embryo adoption, national and international adoption, fostering with intent to adopt, surrogacy, and choosing to remain childless. We discuss the advantages and disadvantages of each option as well as questions you may ask that can assist the hero in choosing the option that is best for them. Let's start with fertility treatments.

Fertility Treatments

Some people don't pursue fertility treatments due to financial, religious, or ethical reasons. However, for those who do seek medical intervention, many options exist ranging from medications to surgeries. There are advantages and disadvantages related to every type of treatment. For example, fertility drugs can be one of the first lines of treatment, and some of them are relatively inexpensive. But they can cause side effects like bloating, mood swings, and the risk of multiples. In addition, some may be more costly, especially those that are injectable. As mentioned in Chapter 2, intrauterine insemination, in vitro fertilization, gamete intrafallopian transfer, zygote intrafallopian transfer, and surgery are other options, but, depending on the procedure, can be very costly. In addition, they can be both physically and mentally exhausting. And no matter whether your client chooses medications, procedures, surgeries, or a combination of all, success is still not guaranteed.

Egg Donation, Sperm Donation, and Embryo Adoption

Other paths to parenthood include using egg donors, sperm donors, or embryo adoption. Egg donation and sperm donation allow at least one of the partners to be a biologically related parent of the child that is born. Using donor sperm is beneficial for men who struggle with sperm production and/or motility, those who don't want to pass on genetic disorders, and for those who are single or in same-sex relationships. Donor eggs are usually combined with the sperm of the partner and transferred to the woman's uterus. This option is useful for those who have medical conditions that inhibit pregnancy, those who don't want to pass along genetic disorders, or those whose eggs are unlikely to be viable. Some people choose to adopt frozen embryos that are left over from other couples' in vitro fertilization treatments. Depending on the state they live in, this path may involve more legalities than using egg or sperm donation. When it comes to cost, sperm donation is the least expensive option with egg donation and embryo adoption being the most expensive.

Surrogacy

Surrogacy involves one woman carrying another individual or couple's biological child. Surrogacy may be used if both the male and female in a relationship are infertile or if the female partner is unable to carry a baby. Donor sperm combined with the female partner's eggs, donor eggs combined with the male partner's sperm, or adopted embryos are implanted in the surrogate's uterus to achieve pregnancy. This option is very expensive with costs ranging between $100,000.00 and $200,000.00 as the couple must pay for embryo creation, egg donation, agency fees, legal fees, surrogate compensation, and insurance costs (Braverman, 2022). In addition, other considerations include the couple feeling removed from the pregnancy and must deal with laws regarding surrogacy.

With each of these options, you may want to explore with clients which methods they have tried or would be willing to try, how much cost they are willing to incur, how long they plan on pursuing the chosen option, and if their partners are on the same page in any or all areas of concern. In addition, you may want to ask your clients if they want at least one partner in the relationship to be a biological parent and about any religious and ethical beliefs they may hold related to the procedures. In the case of surrogacy, you can examine how they feel about another woman carrying the baby, whether to use donor eggs, donor sperm, or donor embryos, and the high cost. In addition, it's important to discuss that success is not guaranteed. What will they do if their chosen path doesn't work out the way they hoped? What if in vitro fertilization fails? What if a woman miscarries her adopted embryos? What if the surrogate changes her mind about giving up the baby? The outcome is often a moving target, so special consideration should be given to processing these experiences.

Adoption

Adoption is another nontraditional path to parenthood. This may include local adoption, international adoption, or fostering with the intent to adopt. Adoption may be appealing to those who want to help a child in need, help a birth mother in need, or who feel they have a religious and/or civic duty to adopt. Adoption is a lengthy process typically involving an application, home study, being placed on a list, and waiting for a birth mother to choose your home for her child. International adoptions involve international travel to adopt children and fostering involves keeping children in the home for designated periods of time until they can return to their own homes. In some cases, they are unable to return and at that time are available to adopt. Adoption can be very costly, and the process involves many legalities. In addition, adopted children can sometimes have behavioral or emotional problems depending on their past experiences. For clients thinking about adoption, you may want to ask how they feel about rearing children that aren't biologically theirs. Also discuss thoughts about adopting children of different ages and nationalities, the high cost, legal ramifications, and willingness to deal with potential physical and/or behavioral challenges of the children they adopt.

Choosing to Remain Childless

Some couples may choose to remain childless. They may consider non-traditional paths to parenthood and decide to try none of them. They may try one or more of the options without success. Choosing to remain childless is a personal decision that, just like the other paths, has advantages and disadvantages. Remaining childless affords opportunities for personal growth and development, career, travel, and a focus on relationships with a spouse and/or friends. However, consideration should also be given to concerns of loneliness and purpose. Discuss with your clients the opportunities for generativity and legacy and potential ways to engage in children's lives in other ways, if desired. For example, this hero may nurture special relationships with nieces and nephews or volunteer at a local school. You may also want to ask what the new future will look like for them. What is their purpose? What is their plan? How can they engage in activities that will fulfill them in other ways than having biological children? This may also consist of grief work associated with the loss of a dream they had for children.

As you explore nontraditional paths to parenthood with your clients, it is important to discuss their perceptions of these options. And as they make decisions and pursue these paths, you must guide them and support them along the way. They will experience a multitude of emotions on the roller coaster ride. For example, hope may turn to despair when in vitro fertilization doesn't work. Anxiety may permeate when several years have gone by without being chosen by a birth mother. Grief may take its toll when a foster child is suddenly removed from the foster home and given back to the family. You can walk alongside them on the journey and ask how it's going, what hurdles they've faced, and what successes they've achieved.

As heroes walk this path, they may encounter people along the way who are curious about why they don't have children. It's a question they may get often on the journey, especially if it lasts years. How will they respond? In the next section, we explore how your clients might handle the situation when asked, "When are you having children?"

TY'S STORY

I never even really thought I would get married, much less have kids. So, when I met and married Zhen, I was over the moon. I had found somebody to spend the rest of my life with. We were living the dream. It seemed like we had it all. Man, we were happy. Until she wanted to get pregnant and couldn't. It was a lot harder on her than me. Having kids was something I never thought about, so not having them wasn't a big deal. But to her? It was everything. I felt so helpless. I wanted to make it better for her. I wanted to make it go away. But there was nothing I could do or say to change any of it. I went along with all the doctor visits and masturbating in a cup and giving her shots in the butt. I mean, I wanted to do what I could to help her dreams come true. But none of it mattered. All that money? Wasted. All that time? Gone. And all those hopes and dreams? Crushed. When she started talking about adoption, that's when I put my foot down. I just don't feel good about adopting a kid from who knows where. Too many children are born with issues these days with all the drug babies and stuff like that. I just wasn't ready to take that on. She was disappointed, but she understood where I was coming from. So, now, we're trying to figure out what's next.

One of the things that bothers me the most is when other people ask us when we're having children. We were at the mall the other day, and we ran into a friend we hadn't seen in a while. Of course, he had a whole slew of his kids in tow. After "Hey, how are you?", what do you think was the first thing he asked? *So, when are you two going to pop out a couple?* My usual go-to response is, "The option is always open." Zhen's is, "We'd love to have kids, it just hasn't worked out." So, that's how she answered. This guy comes back with, "Well, you know, God doesn't give us more than we can handle". As soon as he walked away, I looked at Zhen and could tell the waterfall of tears was on the way. She cried to me, "What's he trying to say? We can't handle a kid? We don't have what it takes?"

I deal with these idiots at work, too. This one lady asks me constantly when we're having children. I keep saying, "The option is always open." But, man, I've got to come up with something else. Me and Zhen are 47 years old now, and we've been married 23 years! We're not having any kids at this point. Does this lady not see that? Maybe my answer should be, "We're waiting until we're eligible to draw social security." It drives me crazy! Why won't everybody just leave us alone?

HOW THE HERO CAN RESPOND WHEN ASKED ABOUT CHILDREN

First comes love, then comes marriage, then comes the baby in the baby carriage. We have heard this rhyme and even repeated it since we were small. Most people are so accustomed to seeing their friends, family members, coworkers, neighbors, and church family have children that they assume it's an easy, natural progression for everyone. So, when well-meaning people ask the question, "When are you having children?" or "When are you having more?", they probably don't intend to hurt the one they ask or stir up negative emotions. After all, if they're asking, they may not know it's a struggle. They have no clue it's a sensitive topic. And they have no idea the person doesn't know how to respond, especially if they're caught off guard. Your client may benefit from planning ahead when it comes to answering these types of questions. Having a few stock answers might prevent emotional outbursts, biting sarcasm, backlashes, or some just plain awkward moments. There are different ways to go about it. The plan may depend on where the client is in the process (testing, diagnosis, or treatment), the client's personality and/or values, the person who's asking, how much information the client wants to divulge, or the kind of message the client wants to leave with the curious party. Here are some examples.

How to Respond When Asked About Having Children

- We really want children, but it's just not happened yet.
- We pulled the goalie a long time ago, but nothing's hitting the back of the net.
- When you stop asking.
- I have endometriosis. That makes having children really difficult. Have you ever had a challenging health issue you didn't want to deal with?
- God has a plan for us. We're trusting Him with the outcome.
- You may not realize this, but we've been struggling with infertility for a while now. I can't answer your question because I don't know the answer myself. If, and when, it happens, I'll let you know.
- We've had several miscarriages and are trying to figure out why. Would you mind praying for us?
- We're in the middle of our second round of in vitro fertilization. We hope to get a positive pregnancy test soon.
- Did you know that one in eight people struggle with infertility? I'm one of those.
- I love kids, and I always wanted a big family, but it didn't work out the way I wanted it to. At least as a teacher I have 20 new kids to love on every new school year.
- We don't talk about this much because it's a painful topic. I know you mean well, but I'd appreciate it if you didn't ask again.
- That's a really personal question. Getting pregnant is difficult for some people, and it could create an awkward situation if they don't know how to respond.
- I'd rather not answer that, but I'd love to tell you about my pets.
- I'm not sure. But enough about me. How was your vacation last week?
- After we've put lots of time into practicing.
- What answer could I give you that would make you stop asking?
- Why do you want to know?
- When it happens, it happens. How's the weather in your part of town?
- That's a complicated question. How much time do you have?
- I've been on a waiting list to adopt for three years. Hopefully a birth mother will choose me soon.
- November 3, 2027, at 8:07 A.M. sounds good to me.
- We're having sex often, so we're doing our part.

- We've been trying for a long time! Tomorrow couldn't be soon enough.
- It's none of your business.
- That's personal. Would you like to tell me something about your reproductive system?
- I'd love to in about 9 months, but we'll see.

You may want to ask clients if other people's questions are bothersome or if they have thought about how they might answer if asked. Discuss how they might respond differently to their parents versus their coworkers or how much information they are comfortable sharing. Your clients may see this as an opportunity to educate others about infertility and reproductive loss, or they may see it as an opportunity to shut the door on all future questions. And this response might change over time with the same people. Remember, every story is different. Develop a plan that makes sense for your clients and their unique set of circumstances.

CONCLUSION

The growth of the American population is declining for the first time in history. One reason is the intentional decision to not have as many children or to not have children at all. Yet many people, especially women, still feel internal and external pressure to become mothers. For those who are unable to conceive naturally, many alternatives exist. These include fertility treatments, egg and sperm donation, embryo adoption, national and international adoption, fostering with intent to adopt, and surrogacy. Additionally, some people with infertility may choose to remain childless. Discussing the advantages and disadvantages of these options can assist your clients in choosing and following the path that is right for them. And exploring ways to respond when asked about having children can provide important tools necessary for coping with some potentially uncomfortable situations. It may sometimes feel like the journey is long and will never reach a happy ending, but with your guidance and support, our heroes can successfully rewrite their stories and complete the quest victoriously.

REFERENCES

Atlantic Starr (1987). Always [Song]. On *All in the name of love*. Warner Brothers.

Bernardi, L., & Klarner, A. (2014). Social networks and fertility. *Demographic Research*, *30*(22), 641–670.

Bolick, K. (2016). *Spinster: Making a life of one's own*. Crown.

Braverman, B. (2022). *How much surrogacy costs and how to pay for it*. U.S. News and World Report. https://money.usnews.com/money/personal-finance/family-finance/articles/how-much-surrogacy-costs-and-how-to-pay-for-it#:~:text=Experts%20say%20the%20total%20cost%20can%20range%20from%20%20%24100%2C000%20to%20%24200%2C000.&text=June%202%2C%202022%2C%20at%2010%3A48%20a.m.&text=Many%20would%2Dbe%20parents%20feel,world%20is%20a%20priceless%20experience.

Brown, A. (2021). *Growing share of childless adults in U.S. don't expect to ever have children*. Pew Research Center. https://www.pewresearch.org/fact-tank/2021/11/19/growing-share-of-childless-adults-in-u-s-dont-expect-to-ever-have-children/

Daum, M. (Ed.). (2015). *Selfish, shallow, and self-absorbed: Sixteen writers on the decision not to have kids*. Picador.

Heaton, T.B. (1998). Religious influences on Mormon fertility: Cross-national comparisons. In J.T. Duke (Ed.) *Latter-day saint social life: Social research on the LDS church and its Members* (pp. 425–440). Brigham Young University.

Hoffower, H. (2022). *5 reasons more millennials are choosing not to have children*. Business Insider. https://www.businessinsider.com/why-millennials-birth-fertility-ratedeclining-fewer-babies-2022-1

Ingraham, C. (2015). *Charted: The religions that make the most babies*. The Washington Post. https://www.washingtonpost.com/news/wonk/wp/2015/05/12/charted-the-religions-that-make-the-most-babies/

Lee, R., & Mason A. (2014). Is low fertility really a problem? Population aging, dependency, and consumption. *Science*, *346*(6206), 229–234.

Merriam-Webster (n.d.). *Pronatalist*. Retrieved September 29, 2022, from https://www.merriam-webster.com/dictionary/pronatalist

Orth, T. (2022). *Does society pressure men and women to have children?* YouGovAmerica. https://today.yougov.com/topics/politics/articles-reports/2022/02/08/does-society-pressure-men-and-women-have-children

Pew Research Center (2021, April 7). *Social media fact sheet*. https://www.pewresearch.org/internet/fact-sheet/social-media/

Rogers, L. (2021). *COVID-19, declining birth rates and international migration resulted in historically small population gains*. United States Census Bureau. https://www.census.gov/library/stories/2021/12/us-population-grew-in-2021-slowest-rate-since-founding-of-the-nation.html

Shechter, T. (2019). *A brief history of bullying women to have babies*. Bunk. https://www.bunkhistory.org/resources/4203

Stone, L. (2020). *Pro-natal policies work, but they come with a hefty price tag*. Institute for Family Studies. https://ifstudies.org/blog/pro-natal-policies-work-but-they-come-with-a-hefty-price-tag

United Nations Department of Economics and Social Affairs (2020). *World fertility and family planning 2020: Highlights*. https://www.un.org/en/development/desa/population/publications/pdf/family/World_Fertility_and_Family_Planning_2020_Highlights.pdf

CHAPTER TEN

Multicultural Considerations

Is Infertility an Equal Opportunity Condition?

Infertility. It's not just for the 1950s housewife …

With the idyllic single-income, married, heterosexual couple with 2.5 children and a white picket fence in our rear-view mirror, we have evolved to a broader definition of the American family. Infertility and reproductive loss are indiscriminate, impacting individuals across regions, cultures, and ethnicities. Our attempt to research the diagnostic likelihood of varying infertility diagnoses among different cultures, religions, and races resulted in little data. Searches of the Centers for Disease Control and National Institutes of Health failed to identify stratified data related to which groups are more likely to suffer from infertility. Instead of data supporting varying degrees of infertility diagnoses among groups, our searches unearthed stratified accessibility to treatment outcomes and correlations between power and success in fertility treatments, pointing to the value of addressing these concepts when working with those struggling with infertility.

As helping professionals, specifically counselors, you are ethically mandated to counsel with cultural competency (American Counseling Association, 2014). Although those suffering from infertility and reproductive loss often have many shared experiences, these experiences are colored through the lens through which our hero sees the world and how the world sees them. As helping professionals, you are charged with the difficult task of layering the issue of infertility with our hero's personal characteristics. Throughout Chapter 10, we will systematically explore our hero through the lens of the RESPECTFUL model.

DOI: 10.4324/9781003336402-13

THE RESPECTFUL MODEL

The importance of multicultural awareness for helping professionals first emerged in the 1980s (Ponterotto, 1996). Since then, professional counseling and social work educational programs routinely integrate multicultural counseling into their curriculum, with some courses devoted entirely to cultural competencies. Helping professionals often use structured ways for the practitioner to ensure they recognize and address all aspects of their client's self. The RESPECTFUL Model was introduced in the late 1990s as a strategic, sequential way for helping professionals to see the world in which clients' experiences are shaped by their multifaceted identities.

Throughout Chapter 10, you will learn how the Hero's Journey occurs, with deliberate awareness of how their characteristics shape this process. We will sequentially process through the RESPECTFUL Model (D'Andrea & Daniels, 1997, 2001), addressing the components of our hero's self, with the evaluation of the ten individual cultural considerations outlined in the model. These factors include religion, economic status, sexual identity, psychological maturity, ethnic identity, chronological development, trauma history, family, unique physical characteristics, location of residence, and language barriers. The model is rooted in privilege and power associated with these characteristics and how they permeate many aspects of our clients' lives with far-reaching effects. Helping professionals use this model to gain insight into the relevance of these factors to our Hero's Journey, allowing us to see additional barriers that may exist for some experiencing reproductive loss. We will explore the prevalence of infertility and reproductive loss across populations and explore ways in which you as the helping professional can provide culturally competent care to our hero.

Religion/Spiritual Identity

The initial R of the RESPECTFUL model requires that we consider the client's religion when grappling with any emotionally charged issue, including infertility (D'Andrea & Daniels, 1997, 2001). Many conflate religion and spiritual beliefs, and these are often perceived to be synonymous, but many distinctions between the two exist. The delineations between the two are established and maintained in different ways. Our hero may have been exposed to a particular religion or set of spiritual beliefs during childhood, and this religion may even be synonymous with their culture. As we differentiate from our primary families (Bowen, 1978), we choose to identify with beliefs we are exposed to (or not exposed to) as children or to choose a different spiritual path or different sect of organized religion. These experiences and beliefs often shape our hero's world, view, and consequently, views on parenthood and infertility.

Religious views often play a relevant role in her journey. In addition to the spiritual and existential support our hero may receive from organized religion, she, too, may find her options limited by the doctrine of the church. While fertility treatments have become more commonplace and less stigmatized in secular culture, those clients who participate in organized religion may experience a conflict between the available medical options and their religious views on infertility treatments. This double bind, having to divert from religious doctrine or relinquish preferred avenues to parenthood, adds another layer of difficulty to the experience an infertile individual or couple may be experiencing. In some instances, when seeking support from a higher power through prayer, one's faith may be challenged when this dream fails to come to fruition.

MARCY'S STORY

My fertility journey was one with lots of ups and downs. It was initially a relatively easy pregnancy, following tremendous difficulty conceiving a second time. I was diagnosed with fibroids shortly following my marriage in 2008 and had a surgery to remove several of them. I knew that they would ultimately return and that my fertility window was somewhat limited following the surgery. After a move and job transitions for both me and my husband, our daughter was conceived and born in 2010 after only a few months of trying. We began to attempt to have another child in 2012. In 2013, I sought infertility treatment and began Clomid to stimulate egg release. In 2014, I had endometrial surgery, which was believed to be the issue. Later that year we completed several intrauterine inseminations which were unsuccessful and then deter- mined that in vitro fertilization would not be a viable option for us. We explored traditional adoption and ultimately determined that embryo adoption would be our best option. Every step of this journey was unclear, with no definite answer or direction in which we should go. I found myself second guessing every decision. I sought counsel from a priest at my church and was informed that this type of adoption goes against the doctrine of the Catholic Church. He let me know in no uncertain terms that this was not in accordance with God's plan. I was devastated. I left in anger and didn't return. I felt that the organization in place to help and support me as an individual as well as a family had abandoned me. I implanted and conceived my twin boys through embryo adoption in 2015. Although I gained two beautiful children, the loss of my faith and support system has been profound.

Economic Class Background

The "E" in the RESPECTFUL Model refers to economics or socio-economic status. Societal norms related to women struggling with infertility often exclude the poor. Impoverished women are often pigeonholed as fertile and unlikely to struggle with the difficulties associated with infertility (Bell, 2009). Beyond the stereotype of being highly fertile, barriers associated with seeking alternative means of becoming parents exist for those with low socio-economic status. The average cost of completing a series of medical fertility treatments in 2011 ranged from $1,182 (for less expensive, less invasive hormonal treatments) to nearly $61,337 for multiple in vitro fertilization cycles (Katz et al., 2011). A June 2022 Forbes report dissected the costs associated with each component of fertility treatment, with base fees for a single fresh egg retrieval nearing the $50,000 dollar mark and surrogacy topping $150,000 (Conrad & Grifo, 2022). While the exact cost of assisted reproductive technology varies based on several factors, these numbers indicate the substantial financial barriers associated with treatments for infertility.

In some instances, insurance will cover some or all of infertility treatments, depending on the insurance plan and state legislature. However, this benefit is only available to those who have health insurance benefits accompanying their position, excluding a large portion of the population. The costs associated with fertility treatments and adoption are so prohibitive that it is unlikely anyone near or around the poverty line, or even those who are middle class, could afford them without supplements. Let's compare some numbers. According to the Child Welfare Information Gateway (2022), the cost of an independent adoption ranges from $15,000 to $40,000. The poverty line varies state by state but generally falls between an annual income of $19,000–$25,000 for a family of two with middle-class incomes ranging from $52,200 to $156,600 for a family of three (Snider & Kerr, 2022). These numbers illustrate how unreachable fertility treatments are to poor and even middle-class Americans. These financial limitations are likely to add additional stress to individuals struggling with infertility and reproductive loss. Knowing that opportunities to conceive exist and might possibly result in children but are out of reach may amplify feelings of grief and anger already associated with infertility.

Sexual Identity

The "S" in the RESPECTFUL Model refers to sexual identity. "I just don't have the right plumbing" is how one of the individuals interviewed for this book described the physical limitations associated with conception with her same-sex partner. The legalization of gay marriage has only been in effect since the mid-2010s (*Obergefell v. Hodges*, 2015), illustrating the barriers homosexual couples face when attempting to build their families. Until recently, even a family of two was not legally recognized. While societal views on gay and lesbian couples becoming parents seem to have softened, homosexual couples are still faced with intolerance when seeking parenthood (Goldberg & Smith, 2011). Individuals attuned to their sexuality at an early age have the secondary realization that their sexual preference is incompatible with parenthood, at least through traditional means.

The Centers for Disease Control and Prevention's definition of infertility is an inability to conceive following a year of regular sex (2022). By this definition, approximately 19% of women (Centers for Disease Control and Prevention, 2022) and 10% of men (Cleveland Clinic, 2021) experience infertility. These definitions of infertility are exclusionary, only accounting for those engaged in heterosexual sex. In Chapter 2, we introduced more recent and inclusive definitions of infertility. In 2019, The American College of Obstetricians and Gynecologists shifted their diagnosis to include failure to achieve pregnancy within 12 months of unprotected intercourse *or* therapeutic donor insemination in women younger than 35 years or within six months in women older than 35 years. The use of more inclusionary terms may allow diagnostic factors to include non-heterosexual couples.

Despite this change, it is of note that not every medical resource or insurance company has a shared consensus on these definitions. These definitions are integral to medical diagnosis and subsequent insurance coverage for the treatment of infertility, putting non-heterosexual and single individuals at a disadvantage. While options such as adoption and embryo adoption are available to traditional heterosexual couples, homosexual couples or those not in an intimate partnership may also be excluded from these alternatives. The Movement Advancement Project is a group that surveys and reports on state and federal legislature. Findings of their research include that although it is illegal to ban the adoption of gay couples in the United States, state legislatures allowing for discrimination from foster care and private adoption agencies still exist (Movement Advancement Project, n.d.).

The intersection of socioeconomic status, religion, sexual identity, and other factors impacts the LGBTQ population's ability to become parents. Helping professionals counseling homosexual couples requires individualized intervention and dedication to the unique barriers experienced by this population. Awareness of the barriers associated with their attempts to build a family, such as formal legal and societal discrimination, is imperative. Members of this population may experience the compounding effect of being a member of the LGBTQ community and other marginalized groups, resulting in intersectional discrimination. The vulnerability of this population also cannot be understated. They are at higher risk for addiction (Centers for Disease Control and Prevention, 2016) and suicide (Haas et al., 2011), and helping professionals may need to integrate more risk assessments and interventions among this group than others, particularly when counseling them through their infertility journey.

Psychological Maturity

The "P", within the model refers to psychological maturity, including resiliency and mental wellness. For our hero, this relates to the ability to cope with the chronic condition of infertility. As helping professionals, you understand that our clients come to you with varying degrees of neurosis, resiliency, and risk, as well as protective factors. This balance of hereditary disposition and contextual stressors is illustrated in Zuckerman's (1999) diathesis stress model, often used in the assessment of clients. While some coping skills are associated with maturity (physiological and chronological), we cannot assume that aging is accompanied by psychological maturity. Acknowledgment of psychological maturity reminds the helping professional to be cognizant of the varying personal experiences and reactions of individuals coping with infertility and reproductive loss.

As helping professionals, you must know an individual's baseline functioning, truly a parallel to the concept of psychological maturity. Is our hero suffering from chronic mental health issues upon diagnosis of infertility? Does she have a formal mental health diagnosis? Does she lack distress tolerance or interpersonal effectiveness? While the Global Assessment of Functioning Scale became obsolete with the advent of the DSM-V (American Psychiatric Association, 2013), helping professionals have traditionally based treatment interventions and client expectations on current functionality. The development of a truly individualized support system for our hero must be rooted in assessing current functioning, predisposition and history of mood disorders, tendency towards maladaptive means of coping (substance use and abuse), and even previous experiences with a helping professional.

Ethnic Identity

The "E" addresses ethnic identity. Our hero's ethnicity may be highly relevant in their infertility journey. It is necessary that you, the helping professional, understand the experiences of those struggling with infertility, particularly within the context of their ethnic identity. Caricatures of ethnic minorities still permeate societal views today through images of the endlessly fertile welfare queen, the unfit mother, and the crackhead. These stereotypical views of women of color echo the ramification of years of oppression. Data indicate that ethnic minorities are more likely to suffer longer with infertility and are less likely to receive adequate medical intervention than their white counterparts (Moy et al., 2005).

A 2017 study indicated that regardless of socio-economic status, African American women were likely to simultaneously experience discrimination and stereotyping in the medical environment, particularly the belief that women of color are fertile (Ceballo, 2017). Asian American women also experienced discrimination within the context of the healthcare system (McMurtry et al., 2019), particularly following Asian discrimination associated with the COVID-19 pandemic (Do et al., 2022). Middle Eastern women (Abuelezam et al., 2018) and Native American (Smith, n.d.) women also reported high levels of discrimination within the context of the healthcare system, resulting in both physical and psychological ramifications.

Ginsburg and Rapp (1991) defined the term stratified reproduction, emphasizing the value that society places on the reproduction of white individuals above that of ethnic minorities. Women of color often experience this value discrepancy on a personal level. In addition to experiencing broad and direct marginalization, women of color are more likely to self-isolate, neglecting to reach out for support from family and friends, perhaps even creating hesitancy for seeking counseling (Ceballo, 2017). This hesitancy is often amplified by the lack of helping professionals who share their ethnic backgrounds. Multicultural competency remains an ethical mandate but helping professionals often fall short in the expression of empathy to clients and people of color (Fitzgerald, 2018). This combination of substandard medical care and a lack of proper support only adds to the difficulties experienced by infertile women with a marginalized ethnic status.

SHARON'S STORY

You just don't talk about infertility. It is not an issue. We expect that we (Latina women) are going to be very fertile and that we will have no problem having kids. As a first generation immigrant, I focused on getting a college education, having a good job, and making enough money so I would not have the same struggles as my parents. My family didn't talk about fertility issues. My friends were not thinking about it. It was not a thing.

I had two miscarriages in my early forties and realized that carrying a pregnancy was going to be a problem for me. By that time, unfortunately, I had left liberal Massachusetts, where fertility treatments would have been covered and had moved to Tennessee/the south where health care services are much more limited as is health insurance coverage. My options for treatment were very limited in Tennessee, and I did not have the time nor resources to try to seek assistance out of state. I went to a provider who was highly recommended by several individuals and my primary care physician. I am Dominican and my husband is Jamaican. We dress up for medical appointments to try to avoid any implicit biases about who we are and our ability to understand the process or our ability to pay for treatments. From the moment that we met with the provider, he focused on the cost of the procedures, although we had never raised it as an issue or given any indication that it would have been a problem.

After the fertility doctor described every possible option, he would stop and see if this was more expensive than I could afford, that this option cost more than the last option, or this is the most expensive option. Again, we never mentioned that money was a problem. I quickly let him know that I was a professor, and my husband also had a professional position. He then started to ask questions about how long we had been married. They would not provide egg adoption or embryo adoption services for anyone who had not been married for at least three years. This was shocking to us, especially since we had nothing on the paperwork where they had asked how long we had been married. And nowhere did it mention that we had to have been married for a minimum amount of time to receive any of the services.

The doctor then refused to do any genetic testing or testing of my eggs because he said that I was too old at 43, and the science shows that I would not have good eggs. We left that office visit devastated. About six months later I found another provider. However, because of the limited options, I had to travel almost 90 minutes for most of the major appointments related to the in vitro fertilization process.

We ended up going with donated eggs. The provider used their own egg donors. Because we are in east Tennessee, my options for an ethnic or racial match were very limited. The donors were listed by hair color, which was very odd. For example, they listed blonde, light blonde, brunette, dark brunette, redheads, and then they had very limited options for anything that was racially or ethnically diverse. There were approximately two Latina donors, about three or four black donors, and one Asian American. There were no options for donors if you were seeking or looking for someone who is South Asian, Middle Eastern, or other ethnicities.

The provider never had a conversation with us about whether cultural or ethnic and racial characteristics were important to us. They did not give us an option to seek more diverse donors. Given the difficulties that we had had finding providers in our geographic area, we just chose to go with Caucasian donors who had many characteristics that we were looking for. It was a strange process with absolutely no cultural humility or even a thought about cross-cultural challenges in picking a donor.

There were also many questions that were part of the embryo preservation conversation that, as a first-generation couple and individuals who didn't really know much about estate planning, we were not prepared to answer. These included questions about what to do if we passed away and how we would handle the inheritance of the embryos or eggs. Again, it was a cultural thing where they probably assumed that we have conversations about estate planning and death in the family, but Latino and black families do not plan for those things.

I am still in the process of in vitro fertilization. We just found out that we were able to create eight embryos. There is definitely a loss that feels a little bit extra with regards to not having the ethnic and racial genetics for our child. We are hoping that nurture will overcome nature and we will be able to teach our kids all of the things that we love about our culture. But as someone who is a very proud Latina and as my husband is even more proud, there is definitely a loss in not having the choice of those characteristics in our donor pool or conversations about what that loss means to us as part of the selection process.

Chronological Development

The "C" emphasizes the importance of one's chronological development in their perception of the world and how they are viewed. In Chapter 5, we focused on the prospect of aging and the relationship between age and fertility. Being a woman of advanced maternal age or being part of an older couple and experiencing infertility may amplify the feelings of both self and social stigma. A mature woman conceiving a child summons images of tabloid photos of celebrities like Janet Jackson and Brigitte Neilson in their 40s and 50s with baby bumps. This becomes fodder for discussion, even ridicule, among grocery store patrons while buying milk. The message inferred by the cover of the tabloid magazines is clear – older women are not meant to be mothers and those who belong on the front of a tabloid magazine. Conversely, the impact of these highly publicized geriatric pregnancies may lull some into false confidence about their ability to conceive into their 30s, 40s, and beyond.

While fertility treatments may be more viable for older and, therefore, more financially established women, they and their partners experience a unique set of barriers. An older woman, perhaps our hero, may reflect internally, even scrutinize, past decisions and relationship choices which deterred her from pursuing parenthood earlier. She may experience negative external feedback from her contextual systems that she is too old to be a mother. Perhaps our hero compares herself to others in her own age group, who may be becoming grandmothers, while she still seeks motherhood. Our aging hero may also be dealing with the emotional ramifications of being physically unable to safely progress through medical interventions assisting her pregnancy. Intrauterine insemination or in vitro fertilization may not be viable options for her even if they were financially attainable. Perhaps our hero has been blindsided by her diagnosis of age-related infertility. She may have misunderstood her timeframe or allowed medical depictions of older women having babies to lull her into security about her own ability to conceive. Your clients may require supplementary support in addition to a particular focus on chronological issues related to these unique situations.

Trauma

The "T" brings attention to our hero's trauma history. The concept of trauma has recently been at the forefront of federal initiatives to improve mental health services, beginning with The Substance Abuse and Mental Health Services Administration's publication of *Guidance for a Trauma-Informed Approach* in 2014. Trauma, a trauma history, or posttraumatic stress disorder (American Psychiatric Association, 2013) are highly relevant to the way in which our hero experiences her journey of infertility and reproductive loss. A history of sexual trauma may exacerbate difficulties associated with the process of natural conception or invasive fertility procedures. Our hero who suffers from trauma associated with the loss of a loved one might experience fertility loss more severely than someone without this trauma history.

Trauma has previously been a subjective term, often difficult to identify due to cultural and familial norms. The advent of the Adverse Childhood Experiences Scale (Murphy et al., 2016) has been instrumental in allowing clients to report experiences of trauma and helping professionals to get a true understanding of these experiences from an objective perspective. The RESPECTFUL Model's attention to trauma brings clinical awareness of both past trauma and its ramifications, as well as potential trauma incurred as a result of one's infertility diagnosis, bringing this to the forefront of the helping professional's periphery.

Our hero, facing the adversity of infertility and reproductive loss, may have a history of trauma or Adverse Childhood Experiences directly or indirectly impacting how they process their infertility diagnosis. Our hero may have direct trauma as listed above or experience disenfranchised grief (Doka, 1989, 1999, 2002) during their journey. Dismissal from medical professionals or rejection from peer groups during this journey may also be categorized as trauma.

Lastly, as helping professionals with an awareness of ways in which clients suffer from reproductive loss, we need to understand how trauma might shape their worldview and decision-making related to this issue.

Family History and Dynamics

The "F" refers to family history and dynamics which are integral to how our hero experiences their world and grapples with emotional issues. In Chapter 7, we explored the value of these interactions through the lens of Bronfenbrenner's Ecosystem. In this chapter, we integrate that model with the RESPECTFUL Model in our hero's fertility journey. The individual or couple struggling with infertility or reproductive loss is often impacted by a multitude of systems including family, friends, and community. These contextual factors may provide support or compound the struggle of our hero. The decision for individuals to share their fertility struggle with these respective groups can be a difficult one, and often attempts to garner support are met with unhelpful and sometimes even hurtful responses and advice. Cultural belonging and identity play a significant role in the expectations and internalized value of fertility in women, adding an additional layer of possible stigma, shame, and isolation. Awareness of the intersection of a client's identity, acculturation, and relationships with these groups is paramount in counseling those suffering from infertility and reproductive loss.

Unique Physical Characteristics

The "U" in the model represents unique physical characteristics and addresses the elephant in the room. What you look like matters, contextually speaking. It shouldn't, but it does. It matters for helping professionals, and it does for our hero. The research says so. *What is Beautiful is Good* is the title of a seminal study on the far-reaching impacts of physical attractiveness (Dion et al., 1972). This seminal study on physical attractiveness and societal perceptions illustrates the impact of our hero's physical features. The findings included perceived positive personal attributes associated with physical attractiveness. People want to be partners with, friends with, and are likely to connect with, attractive people. What does this say about the converse? The RESPECTFUL Model integrates the impact of one's physical characteristics into its structure. As helping professionals, you must take into consideration the physical traits of your client, including those suffering from infertility. Our hero may or may not embody societal traits consistent with beauty impacting her journey.

Is our hero too heavy, too skinny, too tall, too short, or too anything deemed less than optimal by society? Maybe. We already know that discrimination based on race occurs regularly among medical professionals

(Abramson et al., 2015). Who is to say that physical attributes may not play a part in the fertility journey of our clients in other ways? Perhaps they struggle with finding an egg or sperm donor that shares their own physical traits as mentioned in the vignette previously in this chapter. Perhaps they worry a specific physical characteristic will prevent birth mothers from choosing them as adoptive parents. Perhaps they are fearful potential partners won't find them attractive, and, therefore, they won't have anyone with whom to have children. As helping professionals, we would be remiss in failing to enter these factors into the equation.

Location of Residence and Language Differences

The final tenet of the RESPECTFUL Model is "L" and refers primarily to the location in which the hero resides or was reared. The experiences and regional lenses through which individuals experience their infertility journey are shaped by location. Location of residence, or region in which one resides, can be correlated to access to financial resources, assisted reproductive technologies, and potential adoption options. D'Andrea and Daniels (1997) divided the United States into five regions: Northeast, Southeast, Midwest, Southwest, and Northwest, indicating extensive differences in how people think, speak, and interact with one another. Within the Northeast and Northwest, insurance companies often have more broad coverage, including coverage for infertility treatments. Our hero might be treated by medical professionals with a better bedside manner in areas in which more value is placed on person-centered interactions. These interactions are typically associated with the Southeast. The experiences and lenses of people living in different parts of the country can be vastly different. Make sure to explore how your client's location may impact their experience with infertility.

CONCLUSION

The development of the RESPECTFUL Model established a standard for helping professionals to systematically acknowledge the tenets of our client's individual self. The model consists of ten areas of individuation, impacting how our hero interacts with her world. These tenets must be integrated into the counseling relationship and your work with those struggling with infertility or reproductive loss. Again, you, the helping professional, are ethically bound to provide culturally competent counseling to all clients, focusing on "the worth, dignity, potential, and uniqueness of people within their social and cultural contexts" (American Counseling Association, 2014, p. 3). Helping professionals using the RESPECTFUL model ensure a systemic integration of multicultural competency while counseling their clients through their fertility journey.

REFERENCES

Abramson, C.M., Hashemi, M., & Sánchez-Jankowski, M. (2015). Perceived discrimination in U.S. healthcare: Charting the effects of key social characteristics within and across racial groups. *Preventive Medicine Reports*, 2, 615–621. 10.1 016/j.pmedr.2015.07.006

Abuelezam, N.N., El-Sayed, A.M., & Galea, S. (2018). The health of Arab Americans in the United States: An updated comprehensive literature review. *Frontiers in Public Health*, 6, 262. 10.3389/fpubh.2018.00262

American Counseling Association. (2014). *2014 ACA code of ethics*. https://www. counseling.org/docs/default-source/default-document-library/2014-code-of-ethics-finaladdress.pdf

American Psychiatric Association. (2013). *Diagnostic and statistical manual of mental disorders* (5th ed.). 10.1176/appi.books.9780890425596

Bell, A.V. (2009). "It's way out of my league": Low-income women's experiences of medicalized infertility. *Gender & Society*, 23(5), 688–709. 10.1177/08912432 09343708

Bowen, M. (1978). *Family therapy in clinical practice*. Jason Aronson, Inc.

Ceballo, R. (2017). Passion or data points? Studying African American women's experiences with infertility. *Qualitative Psychology*, 4(3), 302–314. 10.1037/ qup0000079

Centers for Disease Control and Prevention. (2016, February 29). *Substance use among gay and bisexual men*. https://www.cdc.gov/msmhealth/substance-abuse.htm

Centers for Disease Control and Prevention. (2022). *Infertility FAQs*. https://www. cdc.gov/reproductivehealth/infertility/index.htm

Child Welfare Information Gateway. (2022). *Planning for adoption: Knowing the costs and resources*. U.S. Department of Health and Human Services, Administration for Children and Families, Children's Bureau. https://www.childwelfare.gov/ pubPDFs/s_costs.pdf

Cleveland Clinic. (2021, May 26). *Male infertility: Causes & treatment*. https://my. clevelandclinic.org/health/diseases/17201-male-infertility

Conrad, M., & Grifo, J. (2022, June, 27). *How much does IVF cost?* Forbes Health. https://www.forbes.com/health/family/how-much-does-ivf-cost/

D'Andrea, M., & Daniels, J. (1997). Multicultural counseling supervision: Central issues, theoretical considerations, and practical strategies. In D.B. Pope-Davis & H.L.K. Coleman (Eds.), *Multicultural competencies: Assessment, education, and training, and supervision* (pp. 290–309). Thousand Oaks, CA: Sage.

D'Andrea, M., & Daniels, J. (2001). Respectful counseling: An integrative multi-dimensional model for counselors. In D. Pope-Davis & H. Coleman (Eds.), *The intersection of race, class, and gender in multicultural counseling* (pp. 417–466). SAGE Publications, Inc., 10.4135/9781452231846.n17

Dion, K., Berscheid, E., & Walster, E. (1972). What is beautiful is good. *Journal of Personality and Social Psychology*, 24(3), 285–290. 10.1037/h003373

Do, Q.A., Yang, J.P., Gaska, K.A., Knopp, K., & Scott, S.B. (2022). Centering Asian American women's health: Prevalence of health care discrimination and associated health outcomes. *Journal of Racial and Ethnic Health Disparities*, 10, 797–804. Advance online publication. 10.1007/s40615-022-01267-w

Doka, K.J. (1989). *Disenfranchised grief: Recognizing and treating hidden sorrow*. Jossey-Bass Publishers.

Doka, K.J. (1999). Disenfranchised grief. *Bereavement Care*, *18*(3) 37–39. 10.1080/02682629908657467

Doka, K.J. (2002). *Disenfranchised grief: New challenges, directions, and strategies for practice*. Research Press.

Fitzgerald, T. (2018, February 13). *The empathy gap between white social workers and clients of color*. USC Suzanne Dworak-Peck School of Social Work. https://dworakpeck.usc.edu/news/the-empathy-gap-between-white-social-workers-and-clients-of-color

Ginsburg, F., & Rapp, R. (1991). The Politics of Reproduction. *Annual Review of Anthropology*, *20*, 311–343. http://www.jstor.org/stable/2155804

Goldberg, A.E., & Smith, J.Z. (2011). Stigma, social context, and mental health: Lesbian and gay couples across the transition to adoptive parenthood. *Journal of Counseling Psychology*, *58*(1), 139–150. 10.1037/a0021684

Haas, A.P., Eliason, M., Mays, V.M., Mathy, R.M., Cochran, S.D., D'Augelli, A.R., Silverman, M.M., Fisher, P.W., Hughes, T., Rosario, M., Russell, S.T., Malley, E., Reed, J., Litts, D.A., Haller, E., Sell, R.L., Remafedi, G., Bradford, J., Beautrais, A.L. … Clayton, P.J. (2011). Suicide and suicide risk in lesbian, gay, bisexual, and transgender populations: Review and recommendations. *Journal of Homosexuality*, *58*(1), 10–51. 10.1080/00918369.2011.534038

Katz, P., Showstack, J., Smith, J.F., Nachtigall, R.D., Millstein, S.G., Wing, H., Eisenberg, M.L., Pasch, L.A., Croughan, M.S., & Adler, N. (2011). Costs of infertility treatment: Results from an 18-month prospective cohort study. *Fertility and Sterility*, *95*(3), 915–921. 10.1016/j.fertnstert.2010.11.026

McMurtry, C.L., Findling, M.G., Casey, L.S., Blendon, R.J., Benson, J.M., Sayde, J.M., & Miller, C. (2019). Discrimination in the United States: Experiences of Asian Americans. *Health Services Research*, *54*(S2), 1419–1430. 10.1111/1475-6773.13225

Movement Advancement Project. (n.d.). *Equality Maps: Foster and Adoption Laws*. Retrieved October 13, 2022 from https://www.lgbtmap.org/equality-maps/foster_and_adoption_laws

Moy, E., Arispe, I.E., Holmes, J.S., & Andrews, R.M. (2005). Preparing the National Healthcare Disparities Report: Gaps in data for assessing racial, ethnic, and socioeconomic disparities in health care. *Medical Care*, *43*(3), I9–I16. http://www.jstor.org/stable/3768233

Murphy, A., Steele, H., Steele, M., Allman, B., Kastner, T., & Dube, S.R. (2016). The Clinical Adverse Childhood Experiences (ACEs) Questionnaire: Implications for trauma-informed behavioral healthcare. In R.D. Briggs (Ed.), *Integrated early childhood behavioral health in primary care: A guide to implementation and evaluation* (pp. 7–16). Springer International Publishing. 10.1007/978-3-319-31815-8_2

Obergefell v. Hodges, 576 U.S. ___ (2015). https://www.supremecourt.gov/opinions/14pdf/14-556_3204.pdf

Ponterotto, J.G. (1996). Multicultural counseling in the twenty-first century. *The Counseling Psychologist*, *24*(2), 259–268. 10.1177/0011000096242005

Smith, M. (n.d.). *Native Americans: A crisis in health equity*. American Bar Association. https://www.americanbar.org/groups/crsj/publications/human_rights_magazine_home/the-state-of-healthcare-in-the-united-states/native-american-crisis-in-health-equity/

Snider, S., & Kerr, M. (2022, August 25). *Where do I fall in the American economic class system?* U.S. News & World Report. https://money.usnews.com/money/personal-finance/family-finance/articles/where-do-i-fall-in-the-american-economic-class-system

Substance Abuse and Mental Health Services Administration [SAMHSA]. (2014, October). *SAMHSA's concept of trauma and guidance for a trauma-informed approach*. HHS Publication No. (SMA) 14-4884. https://store.samhsa.gov/sites/default/files/d7/priv/sma14-4884.pdf

The American College of Obstetricians and Gynecologists (2019). Infertility workup for the women's health specialist: ACOG committee opinion, number 781. *Obstetrics and gynecology*, *133*(6), e377–e384. 10.1097/AOG.0000000000003271

Zuckerman, M. (1999). *Vulnerability to psychopathology: A biosocial model*. American Psychological Association.

PART THREE

Strategies and Suggestions for the Helping Professional

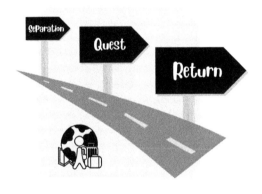

DOI: 10.4324/9781003336402-14

CHAPTER ELEVEN

A Plan of Action for the Clinician

Finding Happily Ever After

We wrote this book specifically for professional helpers who are working with clients experiencing reproductive loss. We know you need the information contained in the previous chapters, but you also need the practical application. How, exactly, can you use the Hero's Journey with your clients?

If you have read this far into the book, you have information about what the experience of infertility is like, and you have the framework for the Hero's Journey, but how do you put those two things together when you are in a session with a client? How you do therapeutic work is unique to you, but it follows a predictable process. The counseling process is framed by your theoretical orientation. Therefore, we are going to walk you through a few of the major psychological theories to provide examples of how to use the Hero's Journey through several theoretical lenses. By the end of this chapter, you may have a greater appreciation for theory as well as an understanding of how to apply what you have learned when working with clients who have experienced infertility or reproductive loss. Both will improve outcomes with your clients.

First, we apply the Hero's Journey framework to the counseling process, showing you how to use the Hero's Journey in each part. Next, we review a few major psychology theories looking specifically at different approaches to the change process. Applying that theory to the Hero's Journey, we offer a case example for the professional helper. Even if you don't find your theory here (because we don't have space to review them all), you'll find examples that guide you on how to integrate theory with this specific journey framework. If you want to review those more in-depth, refer back to the Introduction where we explain each stage of the Hero's Journey. At the end of the chapter, you will also find a brief section on wellness and self-care, which is part of every hero's journey.

DOI: 10.4324/9781003336402-15

THE THERAPEUTIC PROCESS

An essential part of successfully counseling an individual struggling with infertility is understanding the therapeutic process, knowing where the client is in the process, and navigating the client through it. All counselors in training take a skills class to learn this information. Hackney and Cormier (2018) described this process in five stages: relationship building, assessment and diagnosis, goal setting, interventions, and termination/follow-up. They have also added a sixth stage of research and evaluation. In their previous edition of the book, they showed the process as a linear one, but in the 2018 edition, they presented it as cyclical. What they explained to new practitioners is that the therapeutic process follows clear stages, but a skilled counselor recognizes that it often circles through the stages multiple times before the relationship ends.

For clients seeking treatment for infertility, professional helpers need a solid understanding of the counseling process and how their theory and setting inform the process. We expanded Hackney and Cormier's (2018) model to conceptualize the therapeutic process in seven stages, cycling through the middle five stages as often as needed before ending. The seven stages are intake, relationship building, assessment, goal setting, treatment options, evaluating progress, and ending. See Figure 11.1.

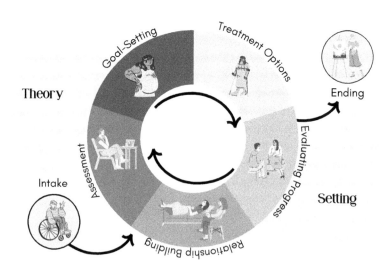

FIGURE 11.1 The Counseling Process for Infertility

In addition to the characteristics of the counselor, two things influence what this process actually looks like in therapy. These are the therapist's theoretical orientation and the agency or setting where the therapy happens. This means that the counseling process may look very different with different practitioners and in different places, yet it will still go through a predictable process.

Theoretical orientation is the net for capturing important information and making sense of it. Your theory may prioritize thoughts, emotions, or behaviors, so those are the things you will look for in verbal and nonverbal communication. Your theory also helps you understand how change occurs which informs which techniques to try. We'll come back to this more in the next section.

The setting will have protocols, procedures, and expectations which also influence the therapeutic process. Some may require extensive formal assessments, and some may encourage creative approaches ... or they could integrate both. Some may dictate the number of sessions available to do the work, while others may be more open-ended. Some may be associated with a religious group or specialize in a specific treatment. Therefore, it is important to recognize how the setting impacts the process. With that in mind, let's look at each stage of the therapeutic process.

Intake

Intake is the introductory portion of therapy. This is when you gather information from the client, provide written informed consent, learn why the client is seeking services, possibly conduct assessments and screenings, and explain billing. Depending on the setting, the assigned counselor may or may not be the one to provide the intake interview.

For most clients, the Separation Phase of the Hero's Journey happens before they seek help, which makes sense since the pain and discomfort from infertility create the need for the client to embark on the journey. Some of this information will be helpful to learn during the intake. You can ask about physical infertility concerns during the medical portion as well as about any medical diagnoses. Ask about any crises or critical events such as miscarriage, tubal pregnancy, or stillbirths. List the main characters in the story and any guides that may have appeared. During the intake, look for an overview of the story, breadth rather than depth. For those clients who do not identify infertility as the presenting problem during intake, you may need to come back and gather this information later.

Relationship Building

Relationship building begins with the first greeting of the therapist and client. It is another phrase to describe the establishment of a therapeutic working relationship. Trust is essential for beneficial therapy, so the counselor must convey trustworthiness through words and actions from the first session. Safety is also imperative for the client to express complicated emotions. The core conditions of empathy, genuineness, and unconditional positive regard are fundamental characteristics of relationship building. If at any point therapy seems to stagnate or the client becomes resistant, then return to relationship building.

This may be a good time to introduce the concept of the Hero's Journey to the client and begin to use story language. You might say something such as, "When I work with people who are struggling with infertility, I like to use the framework of the Hero's Journey. If you've ever watched an epic movie like the *Lord of the Rings* or any Marvel movie, then you are already familiar with it. You are the hero, and as we work together, I want to understand your story, the characters in your story, and the conflicts. I'll walk you through it as we go. What do you think about that framework?"

During relationship building, you will be listening to the client's story and asking questions to help you as you co-author, edit, and help rewrite the story. You might aid the client in identifying a guide when she mentions a helpful person, or you might nudge her to label a helpful resource as a tool. You might identify things as conflict when the client experiences challenges or challenging people. People in her environment are characters in the story, and that desire to give up is a temptation to end the journey. Check in with the client to make sure that this approach is empowering and that she does not perceive it as trivializing her pain. The counselor can still use this method to conceptualize the client's story, but remember to keep the client's needs at the forefront. As with all approaches, it works better with some clients than others.

Assessment

Assessments may be formal or informal, given at specific points, or as needed. Theory and setting may dictate how formal assessments are administered, but all professional helpers are continually conducting assessments. Some provide objective data and aid with diagnosis, while others invite clients to explore. The purpose is to provide data to inform your work.

Formal assessments may be particularly helpful in understanding the Separation Phase. Informal assessments may help more with the Quest Phase. Other mental diagnoses, such as depression, anxiety, obsessive-compulsive disorder, attention deficit hyperactivity disorder, and others may be conceptualized as external villains. As you work together, some may become villains-turned-ally (think Gollum in the *Lord of the Rings* trilogy) as your client understands how those disorders may actually help protect her. Her weaknesses may become areas of strength.

Goal Setting

Some clients may state one reason for seeking services at intake but actually have a different goal. We see this with clients who have experienced trauma and who need to know if the counselor is trustworthy and need to believe that therapy will be helpful before revealing their real purpose. Therefore, it is helpful to spend time establishing the relationship before moving to goal setting. However, if your theory is solution-focused and the setting only provides short-term services, then you may move to goal setting in the first session. These goals may be outcome goals (reduce panic attacks before medical exams) or process goals (develop rapport and trust). Regardless, clearly establish what the client and the counselor hope to accomplish through working together and revising goals as needed.

In the Hero's Journey framework, the very last stage of the Return Phase is called Freedom to Live. Ask the client what living in freedom after this infertility journey might look like. How she answers that question will often inform treatment goals. You might need to challenge her to think about it regardless of how the story ends or with various endings. You might say, "I don't know how your story will end, so what would freedom to live your life be like if you never have children?" "What would freedom to live be like if you have a magically perfect ending?" "What would it be like between those two possibilities?" You could say, "Many describe this as comfort or peace. I like to think of it as the infertility journey as resolved. What words would you use?"

The end goal is to arrive at a place of healing and acceptance about whatever happened on the journey. In goal setting, you want to understand what that means for the client and what markers indicate that she has arrived. Then, you might work your way backwards to the present for short-term treatment goals. For example, a long-term treatment goal might be to grow with her partner to reasonably do what they can to conceive and contentedly accept what happens. A short-term goal would be to research the options and costs of medically assisted conception.

Treatment Options

Once you have established a good working relationship, assessed the client's needs and desires, and determined the treatment goals, the next step is to intentionally work towards them, always informed by theory and setting. The treatment might be talk therapy, expressive arts therapy, a support group, couples counseling, or another approach. Hundreds of appropriate techniques might be incorporated, in line with your theory, to explore the client's story and find solutions. We encourage training in expressive arts to deepen communication and untangle complex emotions, especially for those who use words to deflect or find words to be limiting.

Most likely, your client will be in the Quest Phase during most of your work together, the part of the journey where she is pursuing options to grow her family. This gives you an excellent opportunity to work through each heart-breaking disappointment on the Road of Trials. You can normalize the heightened desire to give up or escape the difficult journey in the Temptation Stage. You can suggest techniques to explore the concept of control over your client's life and how in control or out of control she feels. You can identify her a-ha moments and realizations and identify growing wisdom and even purpose in the journey.

Hopefully, at some point, the infertility journey will metamorphose into a healing journey. Sadly, many clients end their journey when they conceive, adopt, give birth, or decide to remain childless, and they do not move into the Return Phase. This is part of your work together, too, celebrating the quest, but also resolving the ending.

Evaluating Progress

Periodically, evaluate the client's progress towards the treatment goals and how the treatment options are working. Discuss with clients how they evaluate their progress. It may be helpful to informally assess eating patterns, sleep, social relationships, wellness, and any coping behaviors your client uses as well. Evaluate your client's experience with each technique you introduce.

It is also helpful to periodically evaluate how things are going in your work together. This gives you the opportunity to see what is working and what needs to change, and it shows your client that you care. Progress isn't always neatly linear, so using markers in the journey to pause for evaluation may help. One of those markers for evaluation is during the Atonement Stage, when the client realizes that her story is bigger than a personal journey of infertility. This stage often brings a significant reframing of her experience, so it marks a good place to reevaluate treatment goals and next steps.

Ending

At some point, the professional counseling relationship will conclude. Ideally, it ends because the client has received the help needed and no longer needs services. Realistically, it may end because one of you moves, has a baby, changes jobs, or can no longer meet. The ending is an important part of the therapeutic process because it gives you, the helping professional, and your client the opportunity to review your work together, share what it meant, and prepare for the future. Endings are often bittersweet and may bring some surprising responses. Be attuned to your own responses. Remember, you have invested in this relationship, too, and you might mourn the loss of working with this client, worry about her future, and feel gratitude that your paths crossed.

Before ending, ideally, your client needs to walk through the Return Phase. This phase explores how she has changed on this journey and how to reintegrate into her old life as a changed person. She considers people who do not understand her story and perhaps never will. Together, you explore what fears remain and those ghosts from the past that occasionally still haunt her. Help her identify disappointments and how those areas of weakness now give her strength. You will need to talk about her resources going forward and how to find help in the future should she need it. Talk through her freedom to live as the hero of her journey.

MAJOR THEORIES OF PSYCHOLOGY

In your graduate program, you likely took a class on theories. Hopefully, you had an amazing professor who brought it to life, and you completed the course with a rich appreciation for different approaches to helping clients change their lives. If you are like many of us, though, by the end of that course, you had a fuzzy understanding, and many of the theories blurred together. You might have attempted to weave an eclectic approach, picking aspects from several different theories that you liked, but without a solid philosophical understanding to ground your work. That is unfortunate since a clear under-standing of theory helps reduce the complexity of how to help people heal from painful experiences. If you have ever felt overwhelmed by how to help clients and which part of their stories to focus on, you probably lacked the-oretical grounding. Theory gives you a net for catching all the important information that your client is giving you verbally and nonverbally and knowing what information is less important. It guides you about the role of thoughts, feelings, and behavior and how to facilitate change. It also informs your views of development. While most theories are equally effective, you have better treatment outcomes when you identify with a theory. Do you know yours? If you have not found your preferred theory yet, take this as a gentle nudge to pick one.

Obviously, we cannot teach an entire course in psychological theories in one chapter. Given that hundreds of different theories exist (although almost all fit into 12 major theoretical families) we will be making some broad gen-eralizations. However, by using a few of the dozen major theories as examples, we will show you how to individualize this process with your own clients.

It's not important that you follow one theorist's ideas completely. Excellent therapists often integrate concepts and techniques from other theories.

What matters about theory is that it gives you a clear understanding of the change process and the role of thoughts, feelings, and behaviors, drawing from evidence-based approaches. You'll need to know this when working with your heroes. How does she move through grief to healing? Do you prioritize her cognitions, emotions, or actions on the road of trials? How does your theory guide her through difficult spiritual and existential questions? Let's examine how we broadly categorize theories next.

Families of Theories

The purpose of this book is to aid the helping professional in the application of the Hero's Journey to work with clients experiencing infertility. In this chapter, we want to show you how adaptable that framework is in clinical work. It can be overlaid with any theory that you use in your client's work. We don't have the space to go through every theory, but by grouping theories into families, you can see some similarities in their helping approaches. There are, of course, hundreds more theories that branch from these family trees. See Figure 11.2 for a grouping of the major theoretical families.

Psychoanalytic theories, very generally speaking, use logic to tap into the subconscious and create insight. This is usually accomplished through verbal dialogue which might include free association, archetype metaphors, or family stories. Major theories in this category include Freudian, Jungian, and Adlerian theories, all developed by men who were members and leaders in the psychoanalytic society in Vienna, Austria. Professional helpers pay special attention to word choice and repeated patterns. Those who adopt these theories usually believe that thoughts precede feelings which precede behavior. Heroes are helped through logic, insight, and a deeper understanding of what is below the level of consciousness.

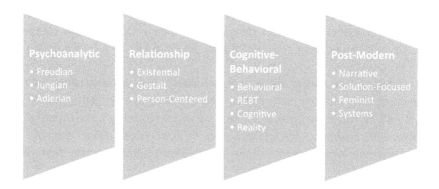

FIGURE 11.2 Families of Theories

Relationship theories incorporate the intuitive and non-verbal into helping work. Examples of these include existential, Gestalt, and person-centered theories. With these approaches, meaning-making happens through safe, trusting relationships as the professional helps clients build awareness through observations and linking ideas. These theories tend to value the individual highly. Those using these approaches generally believe that emotions precede thoughts and behavior. Heroes are helped by warm acceptance of their intuition and trusting themselves.

Cognitive-behavioral theories highly value how clients think and how those cognitions impact behavior in the present. Theories such as cognitive, behavioral, REBT, and reality theories generally do not focus much on the past or why cognitions and behaviors were learned. Instead, the idea is that beliefs determine consequences, so changing beliefs is the method for helping clients. Obviously, those who apply these theories believe that cognitions and learning precede actions and feelings. Heroes are helped by changing the way they think and reframing their situations.

Finally, post-modern approaches like narrative, solution-focused, feminist, and systems theories reflect our modern value for the action. These theories emphasize solutions, social change, and giving a voice to the vulnerable. Those who gravitate toward these usually emphasize actions over thoughts and feelings while recognizing that the "why" may be important for sustaining the action. Heroes are helped by creating a battle plan and doing what needs to be done.

These explanations are very simplified descriptions and leave out many aspects that differentiate theories within families. Theory informs how you approach helping others professionally, and the Hero's Journey story structure works as a technique within that framework. You tailor the technique to work within the goals of the theory, highlighting thoughts, feelings, and actions accordingly. Our goal for discussing theory in this section is to demonstrate that all the theories offer valuable ways to help clients, and the Hero's Journey template can be adapted to any of them. We'll further explain those ideas with cognitive, person-centered, and narrative theory next.

Cognitive Theory

Let's start with a theory that you are familiar with, even if it isn't your theory of choice. The American Psychiatric Association suggested that at least half of all psychiatrists used cognitive behavioral therapy techniques within the last month, and since 2001 all residents have been required to demonstrate competency with it (Psychiatric News, 2006). While the cognitive theory is often integrated with behavioral theory, for our purposes we will explore only cognitive theory, a theory that highlights the impact of how we think. Because it is well-researched and evidence-based, this approach has been used widely with larger corporations and those working with third-party reimbursements (insurance, federal and state aid programs, etc.). It is probable that at some point in your career, you already have or will be using or adapting to cognitive theory, so it's a good one to understand.

Foundational Beliefs of Cognitive Theory

Cognitive theory assumes that cognitions are the major determinants of how you think, feel, and act. It was developed by Aaron Beck, an American professor and psychiatrist, who spent much of his career working with depression and anxiety. Through his work, he recognized that most of his patients developed automatic negative thoughts that occurred so frequently and so quickly that they often weren't even recognized. Most were related to self-evaluation, what others think of you, self-monitoring, and predictions (Beck, 1997).

How do automatic thoughts happen? We all develop schemas, or thought patterns. Beck believed that we are born with a tendency towards certain schemas, but experiences and knowledge shape them. As we grow, we form core beliefs. These are the fundamental beliefs that underlie how we think, feel, and behave. Growing out of our core beliefs, we form intermediate beliefs, which are the attitudes, assumptions, and expectations that guide our interactions. These turn into automatic thoughts, and if they are negative, we refer to them as automatic negative thoughts.

Beck found that people developed negative thoughts in three categories, what he called the negative triad: negative ideas about themselves, the world, and the future (Beck, 1979). Interestingly, he identified that different mental disorders stemmed from different types of disordered thinking. Therefore, according to cognitive theory, the best way to bring significant change comes through identifying and then changing thought patterns.

Heroes have core beliefs, and assumptions about life. A hero may assume that she can do anything she sets her mind to do, or she may assume that she never does anything right. These, and hundreds of other internal expressions, are simply her thoughts, but as they are repeated, they become automatic and are rarely even noticed. When an event happens, such as infertility, those automatic thoughts are then applied to the event. She believes that she can overcome infertility by setting her mind to the problem and finding the solution, or she may assume that she never does anything right and getting pregnant is another one of those things. Her emotions and actions follow her thinking. In the first example, she may spend hours researching doctors and treatment options because her assumption is that she can find the solution to the problem. In the second example, she may sink into feelings of helplessness because her assumption is that no matter what she does, she won't do it right.

Change Process in Cognitive Theory

Every theory begins with assumptions about the best way to overcome problems. In cognitive theory, that assumption is that thoughts determine your feelings and actions, so consciously changing the way you think is how you change your results and how you change how you feel. The goal of this theory is to help clients recognize their automatic thoughts and then help them see how current thinking affects their attitudes, feelings, and behaviors. Next, helping professionals work with them to learn how to change their cognitions so they can live a more fully functioning and meaningful life. Most of the work is in the present, rarely talking about the past.

In the Hero's Journey, you want to uncover the powerful cognitions that repeat with little notice. While she has thousands of thoughts a day, there are probably less than a dozen that are significantly impacting her actions and emotions, so those are the ones you want to uncover. Journaling is an excellent technique for this. Some helpful journal prompts might be:

- If I am infertile, I am ...
- Infertility means ...
- Without children I am ...
- If I have another miscarriage ...
- Having a baby makes me ...

Three Foundational Beliefs of Cognitive Theory

- Thoughts determine actions and feelings.
- Automatic negative thoughts about self, the world, and the future precede mental disorders.
- Changing cognitions changes outcomes.
- Thoughts precede behavior and emotions.

Applying the Hero's Journey to Cognitive Theory

Qwill and her partner want to have a family, but she fears she will never be able to have children. "I've spent my whole life wanting things that other people get easily. It just doesn't happen for me." She began working with a cognitive therapist to cope with anxiety, but a desire to have children keeps coming up.

The cognitive therapist introduced the idea of the Hero's Journey as full of mental battles. She told Qwill that she was the hero in her own story, and

STRATEGIES AND SUGGESTIONS FOR THE HELPING PROFESSIONAL

Qwill responded, "I ain't nobody's hero." "That," said the therapist, "is a thought, but it's only a thought. It's not a fact, even though it may feel like it is. As we work together, I'll help you find more of these thoughts."

They spent several sessions learning how to identify the automatic thoughts that Qwill repeated to herself. Qwill started journaling to uncover them, and as she detected thoughts, she decided if they were helpful or not, and she rewrote the unhelpful ones. She was surprised at how often she thought of herself as "a piece of garbage" and how frequently she had frightening thoughts about the future and the unfairness of her life. Next, the therapist helped Qwill categorize her thoughts. One pattern she identified was catastrophizing, building things up as much worse in her head. Finally, they worked on changing the thoughts, sometimes using data to compare thoughts to facts.

The therapist subtly used the Hero's Journey to reframe Qwill's story. "Sometimes, heroes resist the unknown because they are afraid, but those fears are generated from their thoughts." She introduced 12 cognitive distortions as battles on the road of trials. The therapist also told her that, "The problem isn't that you can't have children like other people. The problem is what you tell yourself about that."

While working on her cognitions, Qwill uncovered the thought that she didn't deserve children because she wasn't in a traditional heterosexual relationship. This thought often was accompanied by a tightening of her chest and a difficult time catching her breath. As she recognized and started to change her cognitions, these symptoms decreased.

Person-Centered Theory

Another theory that you are probably familiar with is the person-centered theory. Most counseling skills courses teach from the perspective of this theory. Regardless of which theory you eventually decide to adopt, person-centered theory blends well with other theories. It places high emphasis on the relationship, which, of course, all therapeutic processes depend on for positive outcomes. Sometimes it is called client-centered.

Foundational Beliefs of Person-Centered Theory

This theory is positive and growth-oriented. Through this lens, the helping professional believes that the client has the answers and the capacity to find those answers if it is within the context of a safe, empathic environment. If you took a counseling skills course, you likely learned Carl Rogers's three core conditions from this theory. They are empathy, genuineness, and unconditional positive regard. If the helping professional can facilitate these core conditions and the client is able to receive them, then, according to person-centered theory, the client will grow in a positive direction. When a client is safe to authentically be themselves and can genuinely feel their emotions without judgment, how they think and act will change.

For clients on the Hero's Journey of infertility, the person-centered approach offers a safe place to explore complex and sometimes socially unacceptable emotions. When the hero feels empathy, witnesses your genuineness, and experiences unconditional positive regard, she develops trust and safety. She learns that out-of-control and frightening emotions, such as jealousy, anger, anxiety, and resentfulness, are cues to her needs. As she discovers those needs, she develops the capacity to meet them in healthy ways.

Many heroes want to be handed an action plan for the battles they face on the road of trials. This theoretical approach does not offer that. Instead, it offers the hero the ability to develop her intuition, trust her feelings, and recognize her value. She is truly the hero of her own story.

Change Process in Person-Centered Theory

The most important part of the change process is a relationship that is based on the three core conditions. Empathy is how the professional helper understands the world from the client's perspective and expresses that back to the client in a way she understands. This is done through reflective statements (which are used more than questions) and body language attuned to the client. Genuineness is a state of being where the counselor and client can both be their authentic selves. Unconditional positive regard is a belief that the client has worth and value simply because she exists, regardless of any thoughts, feelings, or actions.

Change happens when the client can tap into deep, and maybe previously hidden, emotions and genuinely express them without being judged. This happens, for example, when the hero admits that she hates how her body has betrayed her. Admitting this out loud to another person then might lead to the insight that her binge-eating of crunchy cheese curls is an expression of that self-loathing. As she experiences unconditional positive regard, even when admitting what she believes is a reprehensible thing, she begins to see her body as an ally and not the enemy of pregnancy.

The goal is for the hero to trust the helping professional and feel understood, or at least that the counselor is trying to understand. When the three core conditions are met, positive change naturally occurs. Change doesn't happen because the emotion is expressed; it happens because the therapeutic working relationship enables the client to understand more deeply what needs the emotion is drawing attention towards. The responsibility for the change is with the client, but the helping professional is responsible for facilitating a relationship that makes change likely. If change is not happening, then 1) the client knows at some level that she is not ready, and she is correct; 2) the core conditions have not yet been met; or 3) the client needs more time to trust the safety of the core conditions and the helping professional.

Three Foundational Beliefs of Person-Centered Theory

- The relationship is the therapy.
- A high-quality relationship contains empathy, genuineness, and unconditional positive regard.
- When those core conditions are met, positive growth naturally occurs.
- Feelings precede thoughts and actions.

Applying the Hero's Journey to Person-Centered Theory

Beth is a 45-year-old woman who has never married or found a long-term partner. She decided to pursue an international adoption of an 8-year-old girl living in an orphanage with some special needs. She has visited her hoped-for daughter twice already, but the process has been slow. She enjoys a successful career and is financially secure. "If I wait to find someone, I might never have children," says Beth, "and this little girl won't have a home or the medical treatment she needs."

The person-centered therapist reflects to Beth what she says and shows to make sure she understands before introducing the Hero's Journey framework. "I can tell that you are someone that sees a problem and does something about it. This adoption option helps you move forward with having children while at the same time helping a child in a vulnerable situation."

Once the relationship is established, the person-centered therapist asks, "I have an idea that might be helpful for both of us to better understand your story. Would you like to try it?" When Beth eagerly agrees, the therapist explains the three phases of the Hero's Journey, just enough to give them some common language and references. Then, the therapist uses it in reflections like, "That sounds like something a hero would do," or "I wonder if that is something that tempts you to quit the journey to adopt?"

As they work together, Beth can admit that at times she feels unprepared to care for this child's special needs, and she believes that her family is ashamed of her choice. She struggles to ask for help. She really wants to provide a better life for this girl, but she whispers that she wonders if, "my altruism is an attempt to feel better about not being in a relationship." As she is able to weep, identify fears, and say things out loud, Beth says, "You know, nothing has changed about the situation, but I feel totally different about it. It's like it is okay now, and I'm okay now, even with these flaws and not being perfect. How did that happen?"

Narrative Theory

While narrative theory is a post-modern and relatively newer theoretical approach, it makes sense to explore a theory that already uses a story structure. An appreciation for the story is built into this theory, so it lends itself to the Hero's Journey framework well. According to the Ohio State Project Narrative (Project Narrative, n.d.), narrative theory begins with a belief that narrative is a basic human strategy for coming to terms with fundamental elements of our experience. In other words, people already use stories to make sense of life.

The experience of infertility requires the hero to make sense of her experience. Why does her body not conceive or carry a child to term? How can she support her partner with a low sperm count? How can she hold a friend's newborn and wonder if she will ever hold her own someday? Which treatments are right for her? Whose opinions matter? Is it important to become a parent? Who or what controls what happens?

Using a basic story structure, the client is the main character. Her partner, doctors, family, friends, and guides are also characters in her story. She experiences conflicts with nature (a body that will not bear children), with people (her partner, medical professionals, others with strong opinions, those who conceive unwanted children), with society (motherhood messages, peers having children, religious messages), and with herself (guilt, shame, blame). See Appendix B for more on these conflicts. Infertility is externalized as the villain. As the real story moves forward, the main character experiences trials, plot twists, and crises. Narrative theory provides the professional helper with a way to understand the work. It also provides vocabulary (words like story, characters, plot, themes, and chapters).

We have drawn much of this approach from narrative theory. Yet none of us (your authors) claim it as our theoretical orientation, so if you don't either, the Hero's Journey paradigm and its story structure still work. You might integrate some of the techniques and terminology from narrative theory into your own theory, or you might simply use it for conceptualizing your client and guiding your work while staying true to a purer theory approach, whichever theory you choose. Let's get clear on the beliefs, the change process, and the role of thoughts, feelings, and behaviors in narrative theory next.

Foundational Beliefs of Narrative Theory

With a narrative approach, storytelling is an important part of the process. Foremost in this theory is the idea that people are separate from their problems. This means your client struggles with infertility, but she is not labeled as infertile. *Infertile* labels who she is as a person, but infertility is a problem that is separate from her, so that is how you phrase it in this approach. Second, your client is the author of her story, so as she accepts the pen to craft how it ends and rewrites her perceptions about the journey thus far, she becomes empowered to change the story. Finally, as she separates infertility from who she is, she can explore it as a complex character in her story. She may even decide to take what was once her enemy and turn it into an ally.

Change Process in Narrative Theory

Narrative theory emphasizes thoughts over behavior and feelings, but it does not address cognitions directly. Instead, professional helpers focus on how clients think about their stories. Empowerment happens when clients recognize that they can change their stories, and change happens when they mentally rewrite their stories.

Heroes embark on a quest to have a child. They have backstories that motivate their actions and decisions. They experience physical, mental, social, and spiritual battles. Themes repeat in their stories, and meaning happens as the story is shared with another. The journey changes them forever.

Three Foundational Beliefs of Narrative Theory

- People are separate from problems.
- As authors of their lives, people are empowered to rewrite their story.
- Externalized problems become characters in the story.
- Thoughts precede feelings and behavior.

Applying the Hero's Journey to Narrative Theory

Pahla was a 37-year-old teacher who was diagnosed with polycystic ovarian syndrome and endometriosis nine years ago. She and her husband have been married for eleven years, but they never conceived. She began therapy with a narrative counselor to work through the possibility of never having children, though she says she has always wanted them.

The counselor began the work with Pahla by saying, "Tell me your story with infertility." Pahla said, "Oh, I've always wanted to be a mom, ever since I was a little girl." The counselor helped Pahla explore her dreams, hopes, and expectations before she ever knew that infertility would be a problem.

"Let's divide your story into three parts," said the counselor. "The first part of your story is what we'll call the Separation. This is everything that led up to your journey with infertility and what made it inevitable. We're going to call the second part the Quest. That's why you are here today. It's all the struggles and trials you had and may still have on the journey. Finally, at some point, this journey will end. We don't know exactly how, but, as an example, when you are 80, you won't be trying to have children anymore. Maybe, since you came to work on the possibility of never having children, that stage of your journey has ended, but there is still one more part. You came for help to resolve this, so the third part is important. We'll call it the Return."

The counselor carefully helped Pahla separate from her problem. For example, when Pahla described her condition with the polycystic ovarian syndrome as "my PCOS," the counselor gently reminded her that PCOS was a medical diagnosis, but it was not who she was. Pahla learned to talk directly to the PCOS and to describe it by personifying it. She even decided to name it Medusa.

WELLNESS AND SELF-CARE

Before we end this chapter, we must address wellness and self-care. We could write books on this topic (and we have), record podcasts (done that, too), and still not run out of things to say. This is a critical part of therapeutic work both for the client and the helping professional.

We may not need to convince you of the importance of wellness, and hopefully, it is already something that you address with clients. We all need to care for ourselves, particularly in the age of global pandemics, natural disasters, financial recessions, emergency room visits, disgruntled people, and hard days. Yet we struggle with finding time, setting boundaries, putting others' needs before our own, feeling selfish and indulgent, and being overwhelmed (Thomas, 2021a).

Heroes on the journey of infertility often neglect wellness. Sometimes, in the middle of the battle, she must just keep fighting. Other times, she distracts herself from the pain by staying busy. She may do things that seem like they self-sabotage or avoid what could be helpful for a successful quest. Although it seems counter-intuitive, these are attempts at protecting herself from the pain of the journey.

Infertility is draining. It saps physical and emotional energy. Heroes have a high need to care for themselves in every aspect of wellness, but many times, they are just seeking some relief – even temporary relief – from the distress. They need more than pedicures and bubble baths to ease the many losses, so they may choose strategies to numb, avoid, or escape instead. Here is a quick crash course in developing a wellness plan with your clients.

First, recognize what she is already doing that increases her wellness. It is unlikely that she is starting with nothing, even when she feels depleted. What things provide relief? How does she protect herself? When does she feel better?

Second, realize that this current season of life is different from past or future seasons. What used to work may not work any longer, but also what you idealize for the future might not work now. That's okay. Try wellness strategies for this current season of infertility.

Third, look for opportunities for micro-wellness. These are things she can do to replenish herself in less than 15 minutes, which is less than 1% of the day. This is especially important for clients who struggle to find time for self-care. She could experience tremendous benefits from two minutes of deep breathing on a park bench or dancing to one of her favorite high-tempo songs. It might also be helpful to find a couple of quick things that she can do when she receives unexpected news (like a pregnancy announcement or baby shower invite at work) to cope at the moment.

Fourth, self-care is a balance of activity and rest. Sometimes, the hero needs action, but sometimes, she needs to withdraw from doing. Help her honor the balance of both.

Fifth, consider her physical, intellectual, emotional, social, and spiritual areas of wellness. She needs self-care in all these areas, but she doesn't need perfection in any of them. She likely is better at caring for herself in some categories than others. Just recognize that wellness occurs in different parts of her, so try not to avoid or ignore any category of wellness.

Sixth, help her develop one or two consistent habits to nourish her wellness almost every day. This is what we call maintenance. She can then schedule bigger chunks of wellness time every month or so. Habits may not always increase wellness, but it does help keep her from depleting what she has and keeps a few minutes daily focused on the need for it. Scheduling longer self-care activities helps to increase wellness and be intentional about it, especially for those who struggle to have time for it.

Finally, help her realize that caring for herself is kind and courageous. If she needs help, asking for it is a sign of strength, not weakness. If she needs additional assistance, such as medication, she can take it to be kind to herself.

Seven Steps for Wellness

1. Recognize what already works for you.
2. Use wellness strategies that work now, not what worked in the past or you hope will work in the future.
3. Look for wellness opportunities that can be done in less than 15 minutes.
4. Balance activity and rest.
5. Consider how to increase wellness in all categories: physical, intellectual, emotional, social, and spiritual.
6. Develop one or two quick, daily wellness habits and schedule bigger chunks of wellness every month or two.
7. Action! Do what you need to do to care for yourself.

This profession sometimes means hearing the most horrific stories of humanity, watching people in great emotional pain, and balancing career needs with our own needs. Because we are natural helpers, our tendency tends to be caring for others first and sometimes not caring for ourselves because there is nothing left after tending to so many needs around us. This is a gentle reminder to take care of your own wellness, too, because we need you in this profession.

If you want to learn more, read *Wellness that Works: How to Create a Wellness Plan* (Thomas, 2021b). If you want to learn more about challenges, read *Overcoming Challenges: Making Your Wellness Plan Work* (Thomas, 2021a). Wellness is not about guilt because you aren't doing what you think you are supposed to be doing. It isn't about losing weight or ticking things off a task list. Wellness is recognizing your needs and caring for them. It is caring for yourself. A by-product of that is that you have more to give others, which most helpers find incredibly meaningful.

As the helping professional and guide in the Hero's Journey, part of your role is to address self-care with your client (and to model it). Periodically check in with her physical, mental, emotional, social, and spiritual wellness. Talk about her personal wellness challenges and her favorite strategies to escape, numb, and avoid and whether those increase or decrease her wellness. Discuss her social boundaries for different relationships and whether they isolate her (too rigid) or allow her to be repeatedly hurt (too permeable). Guide her through creating a simple, quick wellness plan that she can maintain most days. Finally, remind her that she has permission to care for herself.

CONCLUSION

In this chapter, we shared some of our ideas for applying the Hero's Journey to therapeutic work. We showed you the counseling process for infertility. We explained how to incorporate the Hero's Journey framework into a theoretical approach, especially through different views of the change process and the roles of thoughts, feelings, and behavior according to each theory. We offered a case example for cognitive, person-centered, and narrative theories to illustrate how it works. Finally, we offered some suggestions for addressing wellness and self-care, which is part of every hero's journey. In the next chapter, we turn to the cast of characters to learn more about the hero and those that are part of her journey.

REFERENCES

Beck, A. (1997). The past and future of cognitive therapy. *Journal of Psychotherapy Practice and Research*, 6(4), 276–284.

Beck, A.T. (Ed.). (1979). *Cognitive therapy of depression*. Guilford Press.

Hackney, H.L., & Cormier, S. (2018). *The professional counselor: A process guide to helping, 8th Edition*. Pearson.

Project Narrative. (n.d.). *What is narrative theory?* Retrieved October 10, 2022, from https://projectnarrative.osu.edu/about/what-is-narrative-theory

Psychiatric News. (2006, February 3). *How many psychiatrists use CBT?* 10.1176/pn.41.3.0021a

Thomas, D.A. (2021a). *Overcoming challenges*: *Making your wellness plan work*. Amazon Digital Services.

Thomas, D.A. (2021b). *Wellness that works*: *How to create a wellness Plan*. Amazon Digital Services.

CHAPTER TWELVE

Working with Individuals, Partners, and Families

The Cast of Characters

This chapter provides practical information for working with those experiencing reproductive loss as well as their partners. We examine the physical, mental, social, and spiritual aspects of infertility for individuals as well as its impacts on their partners and other close relationships. Then, we briefly explore more specialized therapeutic approaches, which may include others in the cast of characters, including couples counseling, grief counseling, the use of expressive arts, and group counseling.

We want to restate how important it is to recognize that your client's story is unique to that person. This chapter offers suggestions and considerations about what she is experiencing, but the examples may not be part of her story. As you read the following sections, you may feel overwhelmed with all the complexities of understanding her experience. Our suggestion is simply this: ask your client. Ask open-ended questions about her physical, mental, emotional, spiritual, and social experiences with infertility. Then, pair your client's individual experiences with your knowledge of evidence-based practices.

THE CAST

Your client is the main character, the hero in her journey through infertility, but other characters are also important in the story. Some provide support, and some provide conflict… and sometimes the same character does both. In this section, we want to discuss some of the most common members of the cast, the hero, her partner, family, friends, and children.

The Hero

Your primary concern will be for your client. You will be most familiar with her story, but this particular story is told completely from the client's point of view. It's important to keep in mind that your role is to hear and understand her perspective, not to uncover objective truth. At times you may challenge her perspective, but only after understanding it. Gender identity is a topic at the forefront of many discussions these days, so how your client views gender is essential to understanding her perspective. In this book, we have purposely used the pronouns *she* and *her* in reference to clients to draw attention to some of the uniquely female aspects of infertility, but because each client is different, you want to understand it from your specific client's point of view. Keeping that in mind, infertility impacts every part of your client's life, physically, mentally, emotionally, socially, and spiritually.

Physical Impacts of Infertility for the Hero

In Chapter 2, we reviewed the physical impacts of infertility. Your female client may experience many of these physical challenges. She may deal with physical changes to her menstrual cycle. She may have a very predictable cycle or one that is highly erratic, and it may be accompanied by physical pain. Her hormones fluctuate during the cycle, changing her uterine lining, egg release, blood sugar levels, and acne. She may have a sense that her body is letting her down, not working properly, or that it is punishing her.

If she seeks medical assistance, she may experience vaginal ultrasounds, cervical scrapings, and uterine procedures. She may have laparoscopic surgeries for endometriosis, ovarian cysts, or fibroids. As a result, your client may have experienced the risks of these procedures, complicating the physical impact. Allergic responses to anesthesia, perforated intestines, and infections are just a few of the rare, but possible, risks. Many of these treatments occur in a doctor's office or hospital, and some patients experience physical stress symptoms in those environments.

Some treatment options require medication. Hormones may need to be injected. These, too, have risks and side effects. She may have an aversion to needles or lack any medical training but finds herself required to manage and self-administer a complicated regimen of medicines. She has likely experienced a disconnection from her physical body to cope with the medical treatments. This chapter is not about listing all the physical aspects that could occur, but encouraging you, the helping professional, to explore how she experiences the physical side of infertility. This disconnection with her physical body is especially important to investigate.

Some women do get pregnant but do not carry the baby to term, perhaps multiple times. Their doctors may not be able to provide information about why it happened, leaving it ambiguous instead of providing the scientific facts she desires. The grief may be more disenfranchised if it happens earlier, before the pregnancy is recognized by others (Doka, 1989, 1999, 2002).

Food may become a coping mechanism and way to numb the physical and emotional pain, creating physical consequences from over- or undereating. She may intensely crave highly processed, high-sugar, and high-fat comfort foods to dull the pain, or she may disconnect from her hunger cues as a strategy to regain control. In one study (Richard et al., 2017), researchers found food cravers who ruminate more often about high-calorie snack foods also consume more snack foods in response to intense cravings. This has direct implications on weight and physical health, but it feels easier to think about snacks than grief. Similarly, other things ingested to cope with emotional pain, such as drugs or alcohol, may also affect the physical body.

Ask your client to explain her physical experiences. How regular are her periods? What is the cycle like for her? What are her pain levels? Did she have any complications from the procedure? How does she feel about going to a medical office? How does she feel about her body? Does she experience food cravings related to infertility? What are her individual hormone fluctuations like? How have they changed? How has her understanding of how her body functions changed?

Mental Impacts of Infertility for the Hero

We all have experienced self-talk. The hero has an internal monologue that develops as she makes sense of her experiences. We each think 70,000 thoughts per day, but most of them are ones we have repeated (Cleveland Clinic, n.d.). The hero developed messages in youth that were repeated automatically without her recognition long into adulthood as she learned to navigate life. This mental chatter may be positive, such as, "You are strong and know how to weather challenges," or it may be negative, such as, "You always screw things up," but once she developed them, she looked for confirmation.

Cognitions filter out all the new information and quickly put it in categories, but those filters are accumulated through previous life experiences. Therefore, your client's past will influence how she filters infertility and what her self-talk messages will be. You will want to explore her cognitions about the core needs of safety and security, empowerment and control, inner worth, and value and relationships (Thomas & Morris, 2020) which may be strong motivators for seemingly illogical behaviors.

Many women describe some of the vaginal medical procedures as leaving them feeling willingly violated. They experience a double bind. Because a woman wants to get pregnant and will do nearly anything to do so, she often pays for expensive treatments and willingly travels to a medical facility for them. Yet afterward, she may struggle with allowing medical equipment and fingers in her vaginal space and substituting sexual intercourse with syringes and frozen embryos. This may create intense cognitive dissonance as she attempts to come to terms with seeking out and desiring procedures that may help her get pregnant while trading intimate intercourse with her partner for gynecological stirrups and additional people in the office.

If your client already had a mental diagnosis, then that will be another layer of her experience with infertility. Some women receive a mental diagnosis during this life crisis. One study found that 40.8% of a sample of women experiencing infertility had depression, and 86.8% experienced anxiety; researchers also found a significant correlational relationship with the duration of infertility (Ramezanzadeh et al., 2004). In other words, the longer the hero experiences infertility, the more likely she is to also experience depression and anxiety.

Ask your client to explain her mental experiences. Journaling might help to capture some of the automatic thoughts that are below her awareness. What does she think about her security if she does not have children? How does infertility seem out of her control? What does not being able to grow her family mean about her worth and value? What does she think about her relationships (with her partner, family, friends, and strangers) as she continues this journey? How have those cognitions changed? Does she feel "willingly violated?" What messages does she repeat to herself?

Emotional Impacts of Infertility for the Hero

While the physical challenges of infertility are broadly recognized, the emotional challenges may be more difficult and surprising for your client. Infertility-specific distress is a term that refers to the degree of emotional strain that is associated with an inability to conceive or experience childbirth (Patel, Sharma, & Kumar, 2018). Infertility often brings a hope/despair cycle, and those living with it may develop higher hopes and lower disappointments as they proceed on the journey. The hero hopes that this may be the month when she discovers that she is pregnant, while also trying to shield herself from disappointment by trying to not get her hopes up. Then, along with any physical pain from her period and natural hormonal shifts, she feels the deep disappointment of not being pregnant again. Because of the roller coaster of ups and downs, she may also be confused about her inability to predict how she may respond to things. One day she may be fine with hearing that a friend is pregnant, and another day she may be completely overwhelmed with sadness and jealousy.

In fact, this complexity of disparate emotions occurring simultaneously and with intensity is confusing for her and those around her. In the example in the previous paragraph, she may experience joy for a friend who has also struggled with infertility, loneliness at being left out of the experience, fear that her friend will lose the baby, jealousy that her friend gets to be pregnant, excitement at helping decorate the nursery and buying baby clothes, depression at not being able to get pregnant, fear that she will remain childless forever, and anger that she has to deal with any of it. More confusingly, she may feel all of that simultaneously. That swirling mix of internal feelings may externalize in remarks and actions that are difficult to understand and seemingly irrational. It is difficult to experience such a complicated mix of conflicting emotions at the same time.

In Chapter 3 we explored the psychological impact of infertility including the disenfranchised grief that accompanies an unrecognized loss. Grief is a significant and hidden part of this journey. While the hero fights battles with physical and mental challenges, she is also fighting battles within. She may blame herself, her partner, or others for the knowledge she lacked, her environment, the government, and the medical field as she experiences the anger that is a natural part of grief. She may express her sadness through tears, withdrawal, loss of motivation, fatigue, or other symptoms of depression. Because she may not have a life to grieve, she may not recognize it as grief at all. If she experienced a miscarriage, stillbirth, or failed adoption she will grieve that loss, too, but it may be unrecognized or dismissed by others, especially if she has another child.

Although it may be difficult to verbalize, ask your client to explain her emotional experiences. Although a single emotion rarely occurs in isolation, it may be helpful to separate and explore them individually to give you both the vocabulary for identifying her feelings. Feelings lists may clarify the nuanced aspects of her experience. Expressive arts may be helpful since words may not adequately communicate what is happening emotionally.

Spiritual Impacts of Infertility for the Hero

Clients are also impacted spiritually by infertility. This journey raises difficult existential questions that may change the hero's worldview. She may wrestle with religious beliefs, cultural values, and her understanding of the divine. Spirituality and science may conflict, and she will wrestle with where the power lies to change her destiny.

The American Counseling Association Code of Ethics (2014) mandates that counselors recognize diversity to support the worth, dignity, potential, and uniqueness of those they help. The Association for Spiritual, Ethical and Religious Values in Counseling (2022) requires professional counselors to apply models of spiritual and religious development and communicate about spirituality and religion in terms that are acceptable to the client. Because spiritual challenges are often part of the hero's journey, professional counselors must diligently address them using the client's vocabulary and comfort level as a guide.

Issues around life and death raise difficult existential questions: Who am I? What does my life mean? What is important? What does my gender mean if I don't procreate? Who decides when life comes into being? What does it mean if my children are not biologically connected to me? What happens when we "play God" with medical procedures? Why are my prayers unanswered? What did I do or not do to cause this? These are hard and uncomfortable questions. You do not need to have the answers, but you do need to wade into the murky waters with your client and provide a safe space for her to say them out loud.

Your client may have strong beliefs rooted in or opposed to formal religious practices. Your job is to explore her beliefs with her. For example, if a client believes that God determines life, then she must grapple with why God withholds the life of a baby from her. As she grieves other intangibles, she may grieve her changing faith and how she sees herself as different from her religious identity. On the other hand, she may receive comfort from her faith and find that she becomes more stable in her spiritual beliefs on this journey.

She may also experience a conflict between spirituality and science. Her religious authorities may discourage medical intervention. She may view seeking medical help as a lack of faith. She may trust one over the other but wish it were different. She may feel let down or abandoned by what she used to believe. She may experience cognitive dissonance as her beliefs change. Part of spirituality is understanding who she is within the context of her environment. Nature is a cycle of birth and death, so where does she fit in the cycle? What are her roles? What is her purpose?

Ask your client to explain her spiritual experiences. What do her spiritual beliefs tell her about infertility? What spiritual practices does she engage in? How have those practices changed since she embarked on this journey? What sacred text does she read or avoid reading? What are the spiritual beliefs of those closest to her, and what messages are they giving her? Does she experience conflict from pursuing non-religious sanctioned fertility treatments? What does she wish were different? What is unsettling for her? What is she afraid to say out loud about her beliefs? How has she asked the divine to change this journey? What happened? Does she experience guilt or fear of being punished because of her choices? Who is she within the context of her environment? Finally, has she found support from her spiritual or religious community? Which spiritual disciplines have been helpful in her faith?

Social Impacts of Infertility for the Hero

Infertility changes, creates, and eliminates relationships, and the social impact may be profound for heroes on this journey. With all the physical, mental, emotional, and spiritual effects of infertility, it makes sense that your client will also experience social implications. She has many types of relationships – with herself, her partner, children, family members of origin, close friends, acquaintances, and professional relationships – and they may all be influenced by where she happens to be on the roller coaster of emotions, her past experiences, her self-talk, and her spiritual beliefs.

This journey changes relationships with the cast of characters she encounters. One of the most significant relationships is the one with her partner if she has one. We will talk more about that relationship in the next section, but it is important to remember that her partner is also taking their own journey physically, mentally, emotionally, spiritually, and socially. The couple may or may not agree on how to have children. The most intimate part of their relationship may change to accommodate ovulation schedules or to protect medical procedures, which may seem like external forces dictating when and where to engage in sexual activities. Other people may offer unsolicited advice on sexual positions, herbal remedies, and ways to reduce stress, and the topic of infertility may dominate communication, leaving other topics unaddressed. Other relationships will also change. As friends and family members start families and move into new developmental life stages, your client may be left behind, relegated to cool aunt status, but still on the outside of what she desires. Relatives may loan or give money to help with the cost of expensive treatments, but with complicated, unspoken agreements. Baby showers, christenings, and Mother's Day services may be too painful to attend, isolating your client from some social gatherings.

She will also create relationships because she is on this journey. She will meet others who experienced infertility and learn from their stories. She will meet medical professionals, but also the staff, who are often the ones who sit with her after bad news is delivered. Support groups, social media groups, and church or community groups may introduce her to others on similar journeys. You may even be the one to bring one of these groups together. If you are interested in starting an infertility support group, we've provided a suggested 12-week group plan in Appendix A. These relationships are important because others on the journey understand the experience, often better than those who have not experienced it.

Your client may cultivate new relationships as old relationships end. Whether they end badly and unresolved or simply fade away as life changes, some of her relationships might deteriorate while she is on this journey. Some will become painful after hurtful comments, because of a lack of understanding, or as she pushes people away. As she feels more isolated in infertility, she may engage with others less. Anxiety, depression, or other mental diagnoses could make this even worse.

Ask your client to explain her social experiences. Which relationships have been beneficial and which ones have been hurtful? What are her boundaries in these relationships like? How has her relationship with her partner changed if she has one? What new relationships have started? Which relationships are fading or have ended? How has a mental diagnosis changed things socially? Where does she experience support? With whom does she need to be on guard? Has money impacted any of her relationships?

The Partner

If you are conducting family or couples counseling, then the partner will be your client, too, but if you are conducting individual counseling, then you may only know the partner through your client's perceptions. This is naturally a skewed perception of reality. Your role is to create a space where your client can explore this complex journey of emotions, thoughts, and behaviors, including things that are unmentionable, difficult to admit, and labeled inappropriate. This requires understanding your client's world through her perspective (empathy), with unwavering support (unconditional positive regard), and by comfortably being yourself (genuineness). At times, however, it may be helpful to offer gentle suggestions about the partner experience. This section will offer some guidance to help.

The hero of this journey, your client, is the main character of the story, and much of the story emphasizes her experience. Partners may also strongly desire children, feel disappointment at setbacks, and be embarrassed with medical procedures, but they also fill the role of sympathetic supporter. While each story is unique, and heroes often recognize the partner's experience, part of the support role is to de-emphasize their own journey and elevate the Hero's Journey.

Physical Impacts of Infertility on the Partner

Partners also experience infertility physically. They may feel pressure to engage in sexual intercourse on demand, provide semen samples in a medical setting, and provide the arms to hug the hurting hero. They may experience medical procedures and medications to address their own infertility issues. If the causes of infertility are with their body, they may assume guilt for putting their partner through the journey. They may change their style of underwear, their diet, and their exercise routines to directly address infertility or to support their partner's efforts. They may also increase responsibility for household chores and maintenance as the hero undergoes treatments and procedures.

Mental Impacts of Infertility on the Partner

Partners may be problem-solvers or favor avoidance strategies, but they bear a heavy mental load as witnesses of the journey. While they experience their own journey, they also have a front-row seat to your client's journey. For many partners, this supportive role may feel like a helpless one. Unable to do anything to relieve physical or emotional pain, they may struggle with what they can do. They may be asked to cause additional pain by giving stinging injections, and they may ignore their own desires and preferences to help your client. Their experience may seem to be one of mental impotence. Any previous mental diagnoses may be exacerbated as they work through their own needs.

Emotional Impacts of Infertility on the Partner

Your client's partner may vicariously experience the emotional roller coaster, but they also feel hope and discouragement for themselves. For some, this may be accompanied by a strong desire to protect your client and shield her from their emotions. The partner may encourage pausing treatments or refraining from activities and celebrations that may increase her pain. Partners witness raw thoughts and emotions that most other people do not, and they may become the unintended target for angry flares and emotional outbursts. Therefore, partners may be navigating their own emotions and the hero's emotions simultaneously. Any already established patterns of escaping, numbing, and avoiding painful emotions (Thomas, 2021) will likely kick in during this time as they cope.

Spiritual Impacts of Infertility on the Partner

Partners will also be seeking answers to those difficult existential questions. They may struggle to determine what their role is in the infertility journey as one who does not experience pregnancy. They may also ask those hard questions mentioned previously in this chapter. Who am I? What does my life mean? What is really important for our family? What does my gender mean if I don't pro-create? Who decides when life comes into being? What does it mean if my children are not biologically connected to me? What happens when we "play God" with medical procedures? Why are my prayers unanswered? For some couples, discussions about these topics bring them closer, but others may open old relationship wounds or bring disagreement. Spiritual beliefs typically inform values, so giving up old beliefs and adding new ones could be threatening to the hero or others.

Social Impacts of Infertility on the Partner

Social situations may be anywhere from enjoyable to painful, and it may be impossible to predict beforehand. Some partners may take on the role of protector and become watchful and vigilant so they can remove your client from difficult situations. They may say or do things that impact family members. Other partners may find relief in social situations and seek them out, with or without your client.

Like the client, partners have many different types of social relationships with the hero, children, family members, close friends, acquaintances, and professional relationships. They may need to reveal information they typically would keep private in this partner role. For example, they may be the spokesperson to cancel attendance at a family gathering or explain needing time off to attend medical appointments with your client.

Family, Friends, and Children

Other people in the hero's cast of characters will be responding to your client's infertility from their perspective while also, hopefully, trying to support the client. This may seem like mixed messages to the client. Her parents may be concerned about the stress and future insecurity caused by taking on debt for medical procedures. Her friends may be concerned about the long-term effects of fertility medications. Other people's concerns may seem like discouragement to continue. The point here is that if others are vested in the outcome of this infertility journey, their motives to help the client will be from their own perspective. While sometimes this may be perceived as supportive to the client, sometimes it may be perceived as opposition.

We won't go into the minor role characters here, but they all have their own perspective on infertility, based on their own physical, mental, emotional, spiritual, and social experiences. Those near the hero who has also been on the hero's journey have a different understanding than someone who conceived easily and naturally. Being able to understand that perspective may help the hero reduce the sting of an insensitive comment.

For those experiencing secondary infertility, their child or children may sense the mother's distress without understanding what is causing it. Some children may internalize a message of not being enough, depending on their developmental stage. Younger children may act out with tantrums or anxiety to get needed attention. Some may express a desire for siblings and not understand why they can't have them. If children are part of family therapy, you will want to explore their physical, emotional, mental, social, and spiritual experiences related to family infertility as well.

SPECIALIZED THERAPEUTIC APPROACHES

We have written this book for helping professionals, so it is likely that you already provide individual therapy with clients. If you work with clients experiencing infertility or reproductive loss, however, we recommend that you expand your skills to include specialized training in couples therapy, grief and loss, the expressive arts, and possibly group therapy. You do not need to become an expert in all of them, but they are great options for continuing education.

Couples Counseling

Most, but not all, clients seeking mental health services for infertility have a partner. This book is written mostly from the female perspective, but as we discussed previously in the chapter, her partner is on the hero's journey both as a supportive character, but also as the main character of their own journey. In couple's counseling, the couple is the client, so you might think of it as one story told from two points of view. This requires some specialized skills, understanding of systems theories, and knowledge of communication.

Grief and Loss Counseling

Unfortunately, infertility is accompanied by much grief and many losses. Miscarriage, stillbirth, failed in vitro fertilization, delayed periods, and other times of hopeful pregnancies that turn into disappointment pepper the journey. The losses are almost too many to count, plus they are often intangible and ambiguous. Having skills in recognizing and identifying losses is essential in this work. Naming them as losses to the hero validates her experience and builds awareness. Grief study has expanded in recent years, so becoming familiar with the stages of grief, such as Kubler-Ross's model discussed in Chapter 3, as well as other conceptualizations of the grieving process, is important.

Expressive Arts

Talk therapy has been tremendously helpful to many people, but it has limits. Clients who are processing grief and trauma often find it difficult to wrap words around complex experiences. We process those experiences in our right brain, but verbalizing those experiences is a left-brained activity, so using a right-brained therapeutic approach to infertility may help some clients process it at a much deeper level. Art, music, sand tray, drama, writing, movement, and photography can all be helpful in identifying and processing the complexity of infertility. Listen to the podcast *Play Therapy Across the Lifespan* season two for episodes on each of these expressive arts to learn more about the ones in which you are interested. You can also read chapter two of the book *Creative Play Therapy: Moving from Helping to Healing* (Thomas & Morris, 2020) for an overview of each one, including a materials list.

Group Counseling

Because infertility is an isolating experience, supportive groups of others who understand it can be very helpful and are highly needed. These groups may be process groups, psychoeducational groups, or a blend of both. You likely had a group counseling course in your training, so you know that leading groups requires specialized training and knowledge of group dynamics. Effectively leading this kind of group can be highly emotional and heavy, so honing your group skills will be beneficial. To help you lead a group using the Hero's Journey model, we've included a 12-session outline in Appendix A.

CONCLUSION

Each journey of infertility is unique because each hero is unique. Her physical, mental, emotional, spiritual, and social experiences will have things in common with other heroes, but the way she experiences infertility will make it different. If she has a partner, their experiences will be from a different perspective. Many partners step into a supportive role, and they may ignore their own struggles. The cast of characters broadens to include family, friends, children, and others the hero encounters. We briefly touched on some specialized therapeutic approaches that may be helpful as you work with heroes, and possibly others, from her cast of characters struggling with infertility. In the next chapter, we expand upon the Hero's Journey and discuss how it can be applied in supervision.

REFERENCES

American Counseling Association. (2014). *ACA code of ethics*. Retrieved October 12, 2022, from http://www.counseling.org/docs/ethics/2014-aca-code-of-ethics.pdf

Association for Spiritual, Ethical and Religious Values in Counseling. (2022). *Spiritual competencies: Competencies for addressing spiritual and religious issues in counseling*. Retrieved September 30, 2022 from https://aservic.org/spiritual-and-religious-competencies/

Cleveland Clinic (n.d). *Healthy brains*. Retrieved September 30, 2022, from https://healthybrains.org/brain-facts/

Doka, K.J. (1989). *Disenfranchised grief: Recognizing hidden sorrow*. Lexington, MA: Lexington Books.

Doka, K.J. (1999). Disenfranchised grief. *Bereavement Care*, *18*, 37–39. 10.1080/02682629908657467

Doka, K.J. (2002). *Disenfranchised grief: New challenges, directions, and strategies for practice*. Champaign, IL: Research Press.

Patel, A., Sharma, P., & Kumar, P. (2018). "In cycles of dreams, despair, and desperation:" Research perspectives on infertility specific distress in patients undergoing fertility treatments. *Journal of Human Reproductive Sciences*, *11*(4), 320–328. 10.4103/jhrs.JHRS_42_18

Ramezanzadeh, F., Aghssa, M.M., Abedinia, N., Zayeri, F., Khanafshar, N., Shariat, M., & Jafarabadi, M. (2004). A survey of relationship between anxiety, depression, and duration of infertility. *BMC Women's Health*, *4*(1), 9. 10.1186/1472-6874-4-9

Richard, A., Meule, A., Reichenberger, J., & Blechert, J. (2017). Food cravings in everyday life: An EMA study on snack-related thoughts, cravings, and consumption. *Appetite*, *113*, 215–223. 10.1016/j.appet.2017.02.037

Thomas, D., & Morris, M. (2020). *Creative play therapy with adolescents and adults: Moving from helping to healing*. New York: Routledge.

Thomas, D.A. (2021). *Overcoming challenges: Making your wellness plan work*. Amazon Digital Services.

CHAPTER THIRTEEN

The Clinical Supervisor's Role

Guiding the Hero's Journey

Helping professionals may have many roles, including working with clients, consulting, teaching, and supervising. In this chapter, we'll focus on the role of the supervisor and how to apply that to the concerns of infertility and reproductive loss. While working with pre-licensed professionals and students, the supervisor provides guidance, information, and insight. For the purpose of this particular supervisory journey, we'll introduce a tri-level infertility supervision model which demonstrates the dynamic when one or more out of the triad (client, clinician/supervisee, or supervisor) are experiencing reproductive loss while the others are not. Finally, we suggest ways to help with a more comprehensive case conceptualization and include a list of questions to consider which might be helpful during supervision.

THE SUPERVISOR'S ROLE

While some would argue that we would benefit from supervision throughout our careers, most professional helpers are required to be supervised during their graduate training and after graduation while pursuing licensure. Each helping profession and state licensure board has different requirements, so we'll address supervision more globally with the goal of showing how the Hero's Journey can be introduced and applied.

The helping professions are based on the idea that skill is gained with experience. While gaining that experience, emerging professionals need supervision. This provides protection for the client and the helper, but meeting regularly with an experienced counselor also creates a professional relationship for asking questions and seeking direction. Good supervision is priceless. This is especially

 DOI: 10.4324/9781003336402-17

important in areas where the counselor may experience countertransference, such as a counselor who has experienced infertility working with a client experiencing infertility. Because the supervisor has more experience, he or she can provide guidance on how to proceed, address things to be aware of, and help new counselors stay aware of their own issues.

In the counseling profession, for example, section F of the ACA Ethical Code (American Counseling Association, 2014), states that the primary responsibility of counseling supervisors is to monitor services provided by their supervisees, including how they communicate their credentials, provide informed consent, and prevent impairment. Supervision provides a place to discuss multicultural concerns, ethical dilemmas, and possible countertransference. Supervisors point the new professional toward helpful resources. With quality supervision, the new helper gains insight into the client's experience, increases empathy, and strengthens unconditional positive regard.

She may also gain insight into her own experience and become more self-aware of when her experiences are influencing the client's work. All counselors bring their own experiences and struggles into the counseling relationship because we all have our own hurts and traumas. Supervision is the place to explore this, perhaps using parallel processing to help the supervisee develop more empathy and understanding for the client. The clinician's own reproductive story, whether currently working to build a family or whether that phase of life is over, influences the therapeutic relationship. It is not uncommon for clinicians to enter this field because of their own reproductive trauma (Jaffe, 2017).

It is essential that we work through our own issues to the place of healing, especially if we are working with clients with similar issues. If we do, our own struggles become a place of strength and understanding. If we do not, we risk harming clients. This may be the most valuable part of supervision, an outside perspective to help identify those unresolved areas.

A HERO'S JOURNEY TRI-LEVEL INFERTILITY SUPERVISION MODEL

Many books and academic articles have been written on supervision. For example, just in the year 2017, scholars wrote 100 articles contributing to the body of counselor education and supervision literature (Minton, 2019). These included 35 on supervision, 30 on understanding stakeholders, 24 on teaching and training, and 11 on professional issues. Several proposed new models or extended the work on established models, such as the discrimination model or the developmental narrative model. Our objective here is to show how the Hero's Journey can be incorporated into whatever model of supervision you use, not to clearly explain them all. Given that limitation, most supervision models include processes to address interventions, conceptualizations, and personalization (Luke & Peters, 2020).

We suggest applying the Hero's Journey framework much like a technique within your supervision model of choice. Three common models used in supervision are theoretical, phenomenological, and developmental. As supervisees bring their work from clients struggling with infertility into supervision or when they express their personal struggles with infertility, the Hero's Journey could be a tool to enhance supervision.

Theoretical models extend psychological theories to the supervision relationship. Generally, the supervisor applies the major tenets of the theory to the supervision process and guides the supervisee with appropriate interventions. The Hero's Journey framework can be used within that theory for case conceptualization and personalizing supervision.

Phenomenological models grew out of humanistic research on creating environments that are conducive to the supervisee's growth (Van Raalte & Andersen, 2000). Supervisors convey empathy and create safe relationships for the trainee to grow at their own pace. These less structured models give the supervisee a parallel experience of safety and growth and reduce the anxiety of evaluation and judgment. These work well with the Hero's Journey framework by applying vocabulary (words like hero, conflict, temptation, quest, etc.) and letting the supervisee guide how much or how little to overtly apply the framework.

Developmental models include stages of supervisee development with different expectations based on the level of knowledge and experience. Since supervisees need to learn the fundamentals of their helping skills first, the Hero's Journey framework would not be introduced until the supervisee has progressed to a more advanced level and is ready for an approach with a specific population.

Whichever model of supervision you favor, apply the Hero's Journey framework in accordance with your approach. If it works for you and the supervisee, you can strategically go through all 15 stages of the framework outlined in the Introduction, applying it in detail. If time is limited, then you might use just the three phases (Separation, Quest, and Return), and apply the Hero's Journey more broadly. Both work and honor the client as a hero on a journey.

Infertility and Supervision

The supervision relationship involves at least three people: the client, the helping professional, and the supervisor. The client may be a couple or a family, the helping professional may be engaging in group supervision, or the supervisor may be under supervision to develop supervisory skills, which means that more than three people may be part of the supervision dynamic. For the sake of this discussion, we'll keep it simple. In our Tri-Level Infertility Supervision Process model, each person is illustrated with an oval. Inside that oval is the person's personal story of infertility.

Any or all of these people in the supervision triad may have experienced infertility, and the experiences of those involved impact the supervisory relationship. That is one of the external factors to consider. Along with that, you also want to consider gender identity, countertransference, and theoretical orientation. Those are on the outside of the ovals, as illustrated in Figure 13.1 below.

With each relationship in those pairings, there are overlapped experiences but also quite a bit of the story that is not shared. The professional helper must navigate empathy for the parts of the hero's infertility story that are different from her own, and the helper must be cautious not to over-identify if parts of their story are similar. Likewise, the supervisor may or may not have experienced infertility, but if she has, then that may be part of the overlapped experiences. It will look different depending on whether the helping professional has experienced infertility or not and whether the supervisor has personal experience with infertility or not. It is not essential to have the experience of infertility to be able to provide help, but it is essential to be aware of how it impacts the therapeutic working alliance.

In supervision, the client's story is filtered through the supervised helper and shared with the supervisor. If the supervisor also has first-hand experience with the client, they would also have overlapping ovals.

Client

The client, or clients, is the reason for the supervisory relationship and the focus of all interactions. She is the one who is hurting and seeking professional services to help. Her story is the Hero's Journey, and she is the one struggling through the road of trials. Because this book is about reproductive loss, we assume that she is struggling with infertility. It may or may not be the identified presenting concern, but it is part of her journey.

Clinician/Supervisee

The professional helper, who is also the supervisee, is the person in the middle, the link between the supervisor and the client. This counselor spends hours listening to the client's story and then sums up the information in minutes for the supervisor. It is the helper's knowledge and experience that inform the questions

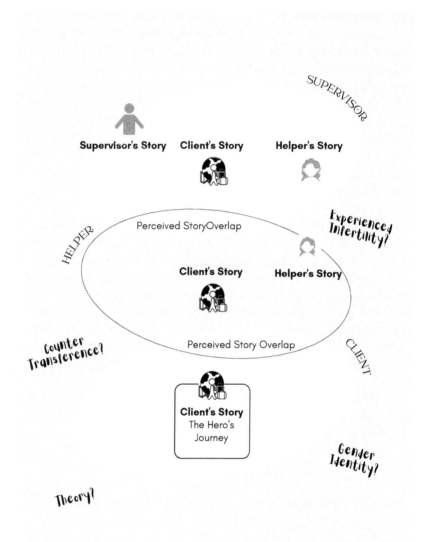

FIGURE 13.1 Tri-Level Infertility Supervision Process

asked, the techniques used, and the theory for making sense of all verbal and nonverbal information. This also means that, unless the supervisor has first-hand knowledge of the client, all of the information comes from the helper's self-report.

These days, gender is a much-debated topic in mental health. While that is not the purpose of this book, we would be remiss not to raise the topic of how gender plays a role in the counseling relationship, especially one exploring reproductive concerns. In Chapter 10, we reviewed the 10 multicultural areas of the RESPECTFUL model (D'Andrea & Daniels, 2001), and we need to remain aware of religion, economic status, sexual identity, psychological maturity, ethnic identity, chronological development, trauma history, family, unique physical characteristics, location of residence, and language barriers. However, one of the most common requests from clients is a helper of a similar gender.

If a client views the therapist as similar to her, she may trust and develop rapport more quickly. The two may be able to talk in shorthand about shared experiences. It may be easier and less embarrassing for a client to talk about her monthly cycle, changes in sexual intercourse, or ovulation with a counselor who has experienced those things, too. While a same-gender counselor might be beneficial for a client working through infertility, it may not always be possible or even necessary. For example, one study of 17,000 students receiving counseling services from 200 different counselors found no differential effects identified based on gender-matching variables (Lambert, 2016). Although matched genders may not improve outcomes, we encourage addressing gender with supervisees early in the relationship and revisiting it any time it seems to be impacting the relationship, as new professionals may not have considered how gender similarities and differences may influence the relationship when working with clients experiencing infertility.

The counselor may or may not have experienced something related to reproductive loss. It is unlikely that the counselor's experience will exactly mirror the client's experience, but some similar experiences may mean the counselor is familiar with the medical lingo, the roller coaster of emotions, and the social challenges. It also means that the counselor has to be highly aware of potential countertransference, projecting their reactions onto the client's experience.

How much, then, should a counselor self-disclose? First, the counselor must be honest. It is always inappropriate, unethical, and possibly detrimental to the counseling relationship to fabricate or misrepresent your experiences. If you have not experienced infertility, you may choose not to disclose that, or you might use it as a way to say, "Help me understand what this is like for you." Self-disclosure should always be about the client. If your experiences will strengthen the counseling relationship and increase trust and rapport, it is probably helpful to self-disclose. However, your client is paying to share their story, not hear the details of yours. That said, we generally recommend brief self-disclosure if you have walked the journey, too.

AUTUMN'S STORY

I sought out counseling services in my own infertility journey. I had a female counselor who never disclosed whether she had experienced infertility or not. However, she was pregnant at the time, and, obviously, she needed to disclose that information before it became obvious to me. Since we had already been working together for a few months, I chose to continue working with her. As the client, it was challenging to talk about my empty womb while watching hers visibly grow, and I sometimes wondered if she really understood. Yet, it also presented some interesting opportunities to talk through those conflicting emotions of being happy for another while grieving my own losses, so I found it beneficial.

Supervisor

The supervisor will possibly never meet the client, and she may not hear the client's story firsthand. This means that the supervisor hears the story filtered through the counselor's experience but also filtered through her own experiences. This could be a strength, but it also presents some challenges. It means that the supervisor relies on the helper's skills with self-reporting, challenges their observations as necessary, and remains aware of how their own biases might affect their understanding. It also means that you, the supervisor, understand the client's story from a step removed, tinted by your own personal and vicarious experiences with infertility. If you have, for example, experienced uterine fibroid treatments as the client has, you may see and understand parts of her story because of your overlapped experiences. However, the client may respond differently or have different outcomes than you did, so be judicious about injecting your own experience into supervision.

Tri-Level Infertility Supervision

One scenario is that all three (client, counselor, and supervisor) have experienced reproductive loss. The benefits of this dynamic are first-hand knowledge of the experience of the Hero's Journey, the perspective from those further on the journey, and possibly higher levels of empathy. The challenges for the therapist and supervisor could be getting too close to personally painful experiences, not yet having reached a place of resolution, and self-protecting in ways that hurt the counseling relationship. It is important to discuss where each one is in their own journey during supervision and how that impacts work together. This may be a place to overtly use parallel processing, using what is happening in the supervisory relationship to increase understanding in the therapeutic relationship.

Another scenario is that either the counselor or the supervisor has experienced infertility, but not both. It's likely that even if counselors or supervisors have not experienced infertility, they know someone who has, perhaps someone close to them. Regardless, professional helpers are experts in helping people heal from painful experiences (even while growing in those skills). The advantages of one not having an infertility experience are that the supervisor or supervisee may be more objective, they have a place to ask awkward questions, and they have someone to alert them to things of which they need to be aware. Some disadvantages are that the one without the personal experience may not feel qualified to offer helpful suggestions or lack understanding of the unique aspects of the Hero's Journey of infertility.

Maybe neither the counselor nor the supervisor has experienced reproductive loss. That is one of the reasons we wrote this book. We do not believe that you must experience similar trauma to be able to help, yet we recognize that shared experiences do often increase trust and rapport. In this dynamic we suggest three things: 1) Do the research to increase your understanding of the journey, 2) Approach working with an infertile client with curiosity, compassion, and questions, asking for clarification when you do not understand, and 3) keep the focus on understanding the client's experience from her perspective. No two journeys are the same anyway, so not having this shared experience does not mean that you won't have successful outcomes.

Case Conceptualization

In supervision, much time is spent on case presentations. For students, learning how to fully conceptualize a client is often part of the clinical experience, and for the newly graduated professional, learning to present concise case summaries with professional colleagues is part of supervision. One way to help your supervisees conceptualize the client's story is through the Hero's Journey paradigm. This could be used as a template for a formal written case conceptualization or an informal verbal presentation. Using this template helps the professional helper and the supervisor identify where the client is in her journey, so when using this for case conceptualization, the remaining phases and stages may not be completed.

Now that you have a better understanding of how a personal infertility experience may impact supervision, let's walk through the 15 parts of the Hero's Journey of infertility and apply it to case conceptualization. See Figure 13.2 for a refresher on the Hero's Journey. Feel free to just use the

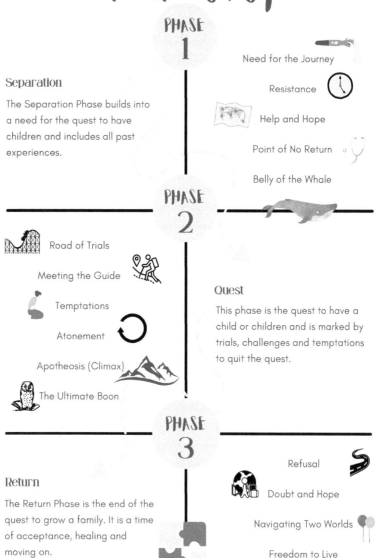

The Hero's Journey of Infertility

PHASE 1

Separation

The Separation Phase builds into a need for the quest to have children and includes all past experiences.

Need for the Journey

Resistance

Help and Hope

Point of No Return

Belly of the Whale

PHASE 2

Road of Trials

Meeting the Guide

Temptations

Atonement

Apotheosis (Climax)

The Ultimate Boon

Quest

This phase is the quest to have a child or children and is marked by trials, challenges and temptations to quit the quest.

PHASE 3

Refusal

Doubt and Hope

Navigating Two Worlds

Freedom to Live

Return

The Return Phase is the end of the quest to grow a family. It is a time of acceptance, healing and moving on.

FIGURE 13.2 The Hero's Journey of Infertility

three phases – Separation, Quest, and Return – for a looser application. Or you might want to go into more detail with the 15 sub-stages up to the point on the journey where the client is. The next section walks you through how to do that with a comprehensive case conceptualization.

The Separation Phase

The Separation Phase details why she is on this journey. It explains why she needs to embark on it, her resistance to taking it, her places of support, her growing acceptance of taking the journey, and the crisis that makes it avoidable. She is separating from her life before infertility. This part of the case conceptualization provides the background information necessary to understand what has created the need to set out on the quest, which is the next phase.

1. *Need for the Journey* – Demographic data (name, birth date, sex, marital status, information about children, living situation, number of sessions, referral source, medical history, past experiences related to infertility, what prompted taking action, etc.
2. *Resistance* – Client's resistance to infertility, symptoms, diagnoses, fears, financial concerns
3. *Help and Hope* – Identify any support, mentors, or experts who offer hope and options
4. *Point of No Return* – Describe client's growing discontent with infertility and her increased commitment to the journey
5. *Belly of the Whale* – What makes the journey unavoidable and what is the first crisis? What identities/labels about infertility is the client adopting?

The Quest Phase

The Quest Phase is the section of the journey that puts focus, energy, finances, and effort into growing a family through whatever options the hero is willing or required to try. It is filled with challenges, existential questions, and roller-coaster emotions. This part of the case conceptualization lists the trials in different domains of the client's life, explores sources of help and information, considers the fears that most tempt her to quit, what she has learned about herself, and how she attributes control over her life. At some point in the second phase, the focus shifts away from getting pregnant, adoption, or other options and moves to what will happen next. If she is further along her journey, it also describes her resolution and acceptance of what happened – regardless of the outcome of the quest to have a baby – and her level of peace with her life.

1. *Road of Trials* – What physical, emotional, mental, social, relational, spiritual, and financial challenges has the client faced?
2. *Meeting the Guide* – Who are unexpected guides who offer information that may help the client? Are you one of these guides?
3. *Temptation* – Describe the client's temptations to end the journey. What is the relationship with the partner like? What are her worst fears? What could end the journey? Even if the client does have children, does she continue to accept and heal?
4. *Atonement* – What answers has the client found about who or what has control over her life? What has learned about herself? What has she determined is the real purpose of her journey?
5. *Apotheosis (or Climax)* – How has the client made peace with and experienced resolution about her infertility journey? Describe this in cognitive terms.
6. *The Ultimate Boon* – How has the client come to terms with infertility and its impacts on her life? How is she experiencing relief and peace? Describe this in emotional terms.

The Return Phase

The Return Phase is about healing from the journey. The quest to grow her family has ended, at least for now, and she needs to make sense of why it happened to her. She may move into this phase pregnant, with a baby, with an older child, without a child, or without another child. In this phase, she re-integrates into life but as a very different person. This part of the case conceptualization explains what has changed, what doubts and fears are lingering, and her resources for this part of the journey.

1. *Refusal* – How is the client adapting socially back into her life? How has infertility impacted her relationship with her partner, family, and friends? What changes are necessary?
2. *Doubt and Hope* – What ghosts, or doubts and fears, from the journey revisit your client? In what ways is the journey not a happy ending? How is the client still wrestling with powers of control in her life? What external resources does the client have? Where is she finding answers? What chance encounters, books, experts, or other sources are aiding the client?
3. *Navigating Two Worlds* – How does your client view her pre-infertility life now? How is your client reintegrating into her changed life? What answers has she found? How has she changed? How does she carry her sorrow and loss? What deeper meaning has she gained? What were the unanticipated positive and negative consequences?

4. *Freedom to Live* – How does the client now experience freedom? How does she describe her healing and resolution? How has she sacrificed her idealism, optimism, and blind trust for wisdom, realism, and faith? How does she describe the scars from the wounds? What is next?

50 QUESTIONS TO CONSIDER

Here are some questions to provide your supervisees in preparing a comprehensive case conceptualization. Since the purpose of conceptualizing the client's journey is to concisely distill all the information known into a brief summary, all these questions may not need to be answered. Some of them cannot be answered yet. The client may not be, for example, in the Return Phase, so those questions will not yet be relevant, and the supervisee won't have answers for those. The purpose of this list is to provide direction on how the professional helper can understand the client using the Hero's Journey framework and share that with the supervisor in a thorough but brief presentation.

The Separation Phase

Demographic Data

1. How many sessions have you met with the client?
2. What is the client's name? Date of birth?
3. What is the client's gender identity?
4. What is the client's education level? Occupation?
5. What is the client's marital/partner status? What is the client's living situation?
6. Does the client have any children? If so, what are the ages and gender of each?
7. How was the client referred to you?
8. What is the client's relevant medical history? Medical diagnoses? Mental diagnoses? Substance abuse?
9. How does the client present herself (appearance, mood, manner of dress, attitude towards the therapist)?
10. What are the client's past experiences related to infertility? Past traumas? Past sexual traumas?
11. What past experiences and knowledge about facing challenges does your hero bring to the story?

12. What prompted the client to seek services now? What clinical symptoms is the client experiencing?
13. What, exactly, does she want? What are the pictures of family that she imagines?
14. What are the client's fears about infertility? What unknowns and ambiguities are increasing fear?
15. What is her worst-case scenario? If she never is able to grow her family, what does that mean for her security, empowerment, worth, and relationships?
16. What drives this journey now? What is the tension between what she desires and what she fears?
17. How is the client resisting the diagnosis or label of infertility?
18. What resources and support does the client have available? What resources are lacking?
19. What is the client's socioeconomic status? What is the financial impact of infertility? Other economic stressors?
20. What makes taking this journey unavoidable? How committed is the client to taking this journey?
21. What identities about infertility is the client adopting? What language does she use to describe herself? For example, "my endo/endometriosis."

The Quest Phase

1. What infertility challenges has the client faced on the journey so far? Physical? Mental? Social? Sexual? Spiritual? Financial? Career?
2. Which of the seven types of conflict is the client experiencing? (character vs. character(s), character vs. society, character vs. nature, character vs. technology, character vs. supernatural, character vs. fate, and character vs. self).
3. How does the client's culture impact her journey? What are her beliefs about parenthood?
4. What coping strategies does the client use to escape, numb, or avoid?
5. What unexpected places have the client found information or assistance?
6. How has the client been tempted to end the journey? How tempting are they?
7. Has the client had children but prematurely ended the journey before reaching healing?
8. To whom or what does the client attribute power over her situation? How has that changed during her journey?
9. What are the client's spiritual beliefs related to infertility?
10. What has the client learned about herself?

11. What has she determined is the real purpose of her journey?
12. How has the client made peace with and experienced a resolution about her infertility journey? Describe this in cognitive terms.
13. How has the client come to terms with infertility and its impacts on her life? How is she experiencing relief and peace? Describe this in emotional terms.

The Return Phase

1. How is the client adapting back to her pre-infertility life socially?
2. How has infertility impacted her relationship with her partner, family, and friends?
3. What changes does she think are necessary?
4. What ghosts (doubts and fears) from the journey revisit your client?
5. In what ways is the journey NOT a happy ending?
6. How is the client still wrestling with powers of control in her life?
7. Where is she currently finding answers? What chance encounters, books, experts, or other sources are aiding the client?
8. How is your client reintegrating into her changed life? What answers has she found? How has she changed?
9. How does your client view her pre-infertility life now? What vocabulary does she use to describe it?
10. How does your client view her road of trials now? What vocabulary does she use to describe it?
11. How does she carry her sorrow and loss? What deeper meaning has she gained?
12. How has she sacrificed her idealism, optimism, and blind trust for wisdom, realism, and faith?
13. What were the unanticipated positive and negative consequences?
14. How does the client now experience freedom?
15. How does she describe her healing and resolution? How does she describe the scars from the wounds?
16. What is next?

CONCLUSION

Working with clients with a presenting concern like infertility for the first time can be daunting, especially for students and new professionals. It gets more complicated if the helping professional has also struggled with infertility. This is one reason supervision is so important. During supervision, a third layer is added, and the supervisor may have experienced infertility as well.

For those providing supervision, the Hero's Journey framework can be applied regardless of which supervision model you use. In this chapter, we provided the visual of the tri-level infertility supervision model, a template for case conceptualization, and a list of 50 questions for some practical ways to apply the Hero's Journey framework to your own style of supervision. In Chapter 14, we discuss how counselor educators can provide wisdom to students who are on the journey of infertility.

REFERENCES

American Counseling Association. (2014). *ACA code of ethics*. Retrieved October 13, 2022, from http://www.counseling.org/docs/ethics/2014-aca-code-of-ethics.pdf

D'Andrea, M., & Daniels, J. (2001). Respectful counseling: An integrative multi-dimensional model for counselors. In D. Pope-Davis, & H. Coleman (Eds.), *The intersection of race, class, and gender in multicultural counseling* (pp. 417–466). SAGE Publications, Inc. 10.4135/9781452231846.n17

Jaffe, J. (2017). Reproductive trauma: Psychotherapy for pregnancy loss and infertility clients from a reproductive story perspective. *Psychotherapy*, *54*(4), 380–385. 10.1037/pst0000125

Lambert, M. (2016). Does client-therapist gender matching influence therapy course or outcome in psychotherapy? *Evidence Based Medicine and Practice*, *2*(2). 10.4172/2471-9919.1000108

Luke, M., & Peters, H.C. (2020). Supervision as the signature pedagogy for counseling leadership. *Teaching and Supervision in Counseling*, *2*(2), 4. 10.7290/tsc020204

Minton, C.A.B. (2019). Counselor education and supervision: 2017 inaugural review. *Counselor Education and Supervision*, *58*(1), 4–17.

Van Raalte, J.L., & Andersen, M.B. (2000). Supervision I: From models to doing. *Doing Sport Psychology*, 153–165.

CHAPTER FOURTEEN

Counselor Educator Wisdom

The Sage

Chapter 14 is for those preparing the next generation of professional helpers. We've all had sage characters in our educational journeys. Some of you are now those professors. In these roles, you are charged with providing education, training, and supervision about how to be a highly qualified, ethical professional helper.

In this chapter, we apply that wisdom to the specific therapeutic concern of infertility. The Centers for Disease Control and Prevention reports that infertility affects nearly one out of every five heterosexual American women ages 15 to 49 who have never been pregnant, and that statistic jumps to one out of four when including those who have difficulty getting pregnant or carrying a pregnancy to term (2022). Considering these numbers, it is very likely that you are teaching students who are struggling with infertility and possibly supervising the clinical experiences for students with clients who are struggling with infertility. Maybe you are one of those statistics, too. How can you be the sage who skillfully guides those you educate?

HOW IS A SAGE DIFFERENT FROM AN EXPERT?

Whoa! I'm no sage. Some of you who are counselor educators started doubting yourself at the title of this chapter. You felt imposter syndrome creeping in and cringed at the idea that you had any special wisdom, especially if you are newer in the profession. Regardless of how confident you are in what you know, your students perceive you as a sage because you are the professor.

What exactly is a sage? The term comes from ancient Greek philosophy, and it means a person who has attained wisdom. That wisdom is gained from

DOI: 10.4324/9781003336402-18

knowledge, experience, reflection, and teaching others (Jenkins, 2022). The expert has knowledge, but the sage has knowledge and experience. The sage has also spent time critically thinking about that knowledge and experience and then teaching it to others. It takes time to accumulate learning and make sense of experiences, which is why sages are more mature. When it comes to infertility, the counselor educator sage has learned about it, experienced it personally or vicariously, has spent time thinking about it, and shares the knowledge and experiences they have reflected on with students.

You've spent years learning and applying knowledge in core counseling areas: 1) ethics and the profession, 2) diversity, 3) growth and development, 4) career development, 5) skills in helping relationships, 6) group work, 7) assessments, and 8) research and program evaluation (Council for Accreditation of Counseling and Related Educational Programs, 2015). How can you now apply knowledge of these core areas to educating others about infertility? You could lead lively discussions about professional ethics around infertility therapy. You might explore how diversity influences access to infertility treatments. You could integrate the challenges of lifespan and career development stage models for clients who can't neatly follow them. You might train emerging professionals in individual and group skills using the counseling process and group plan included in this book as examples. You might guide students using assessments informed by infertility research. Maybe you will even contribute research to add to our empirical knowledge.

A sage and an expert are not necessarily the same thing. An expert is someone with comprehensive and authoritative knowledge. As a counselor educator, you are an expert because you have spent years gaining knowledge that accumulated into the highest degree awarded in your field. In other words, you know a lot. You're the expert, but you may or may not be the sage.

Experience, reflection, and teaching separate sages from experts. You don't just know about infertility from books, even though that knowledge is valuable. You have walked the Hero's Journey of infertility yourself or visited another on her journey. You've reflected on that journey and woven your knowledge and experiences together with new insights. Then, you taught what you learned, not because you held all the answers, but because you knew that your wisdom could help others. Maybe you are a sage after all!

As an educator, you are teaching that knowledge as an expert, but the sage knows how the Hero's Journey works with the therapeutic process. A sage can integrate the Hero's Journey framework into classes with professional helpers in training and provide some clear direction for working with the population experiencing reproductive loss. This kind of sage knows how and when to share the three phases of the Hero's Journey (Separation, Quest, and Return) and when to dive deeper with all 15 stages.

You might not have the beard of Professor Dumbledore, but like him, you will probably enter the hero's story at an important moment. You might directly enter your own client's or student's infertility story, but you might also indirectly serve as a sage who supervises. So, sages, let's take the expertise you have in educating and supervising helpers and apply the Hero's Journey.

USING THE HERO'S JOURNEY AS A TEACHING RESOURCE

We have provided three practical resources that you can use with those you teach. In Chapter 11, you read our model of applying the counseling process to infertility, so you might apply that to complement or advance a student's understanding of the counseling process. In Chapter 13, we provided a detailed case conceptualization to use with supervisees, which you might use in your clinical courses. In Appendix A, we provide a template for an infertility group using this approach. This might be helpful to you as an example of a plan for a group class or a resource for students to use at their clinical sites. We also have case studies and stories in gray boxes throughout the book – many with multicultural applications – that might provide memorable learning for your students. We want you to close this book with some practical resources to aid in your teaching.

While we do not expect this to become part of the general curriculum, as students advance in their learning, applying concepts like the Hero's Journey to specific populations enhances a high-level of learning and application of knowledge. These concepts provide a deeper-level conversation in clinical courses, nice case study examples in development courses, and application examples for treatment courses. Applying concepts with stories of specific examples provides more memorable learning.

GRACE'S STORY

My story began one fateful day in February. I was sitting on the floor of the bedroom with my husband of less than a year in my last semester of school, and we decided to stop using contraceptives. I remember telling my husband, with a sizzling mix of excitement and fear, that we could be pregnant next month. Oh, if only.

We weren't pregnant the next month, the next year, or the next seven years. In fact, it took us nearly 15 years before we had children. Part of that was great. We traveled, and I progressed in my career.

Yet the longing for a family grew like a tumor. We eventually started testing with my OB/GYN, and then we were referred to a fertility clinic. We sat in the waiting room watching news footage of a hurricane and feeling like cattle (herd 'em in, herd 'em out). It seemed like they saw dollar signs and not people at this clinic, so we quit our quest for a few more years. I didn't feel helped or heard by any of the doctors I had seen, but I did feel discouraged and broken. My parents and friends all seemed to get pregnant so easily.

I am a Christian. My faith was (and still is) the compass for my life, but I really struggled to find answers. Why did God give me such a longing for children but seem to withhold them from me? I could have been quite content without that longing. I loved kids. Why would God give me those gifts and talents for helping children, but hold any prospects for my own out of reach? Why were there so many stories in the Bible of women who struggled with infertility (Sarah, Rachel, Rebecca, Hannah, and Elizabeth)? What could I learn from their stories if we never had children? How did being older parents shape their eventual children? How long should I wait? I prayed, yet those prayers remained unanswered. I studied the Bible, like I was still in graduate school, and I believe my answer was the verse, "Here am I and the children the Lord has given me" (Is 8:18 and Hebrews 2:13), but year after year there were no children. I avoided baby showers, Mother's Day church services, and young married Sunday school classes because they were too painful to endure. And the years passed.

Ten years into our journey, we moved so I could earn another degree. One benefit of not having children was that it was easier to go back to school. With a fresh start and new options available, we decided to seek help conceiving again. We found an amazing doctor who buoyed our hopes, but she used phrases like, "If you want this womb to have your children, then we could try … " with fairly low percentages for success. My periods were incredibly painful by this time, and I had diagnoses of endometriosis and polycystic ovarian syndrome, so I underwent my first surgery … ever. The endometriosis was so bad that she couldn't complete the surgery without a couple of other specialty surgeons. Meanwhile, she had to move her practice after a hospital buy out, and we couldn't continue with her. More hopes dashed.

At this point, I also sought help from a counselor, and I found an infertility support group. Both were terrifying to start, had some incredible challenges during, and in the end were the most beneficial parts of this journey. My small support group announced five pregnancies in one night (all but two of us), and I still was left with agonizing periods that came every 26 days like clockwork. (That's an extra painful period every year.) Yet the support and friendships that I gained are more precious to me than gems. These people were all on the journey, too, and they understood the road of trials better than anyone else in my life.

My husband and I found yet another fertility specialist, one who provided services in embryo donation. I learned about this from one of the women in the support group, another gift I got from these guides on my journey. We received embryos from a donor couple who, after unsuccessful in vitro fertilization, decided to adopt instead. For our first procedure, the medical team thawed three embryos. One didn't survive the thaw, two were surgically inserted ... and one implanted. We were pregnant and overjoyed!

Food tasted so good, and I didn't have a day of morning sickness, something that I had joked for years that I would gratefully welcome because it would have meant I was pregnant. We were very private about our journey, so as we were heading towards the first trimester mark, we started planning how to tell our friends and family at Christmas about our anticipated little one.

Instead, after an ultrasound with no heartbeat, I spent Thanksgiving praying that my favorite holiday wouldn't be the day I miscarried. It came a few days later, and instead of celebrating our happy news with others, we quietly cried.

I'm not sure we would have willingly risked that kind of heartbreak again, but we had four embryos left. After a year of grieving and paying off the debt of the first procedure, we decided to try again. This time, both embryos implanted. I was elated, but much more cautious this time. With each ultrasound, I felt such relief when I could hear the heartbeats and then see them moving. I felt the first movement at a Christmas service, and that was when I started to feel assurance that these babies might be okay. Our journey seemed to be coming full circle. That December, at my graduation, we told my family. Twins came a few months later, and another baby followed. Seven embryos, three pregnancies, and two birth dates. Our quest to have children finally ended.

I started my career as a counselor educator, had a surprise hysterectomy, and life accelerated with toddlers. An aging parent moved in with us, and we grappled to make it through the busy days. A few years later, I was surprised to realize that I had more grief work to do around the miscarriage. We had such joy about having the babies that it made it easy to ignore the loss, a loss that was so ambiguous. We didn't have a funeral or even a gender for the baby we lost. The baby had been due on my mother-in-law's birthday, and we'd lost her, too. It all seemed so complicated, and back in the present, I was gradually losing a parent to dementia, mixing in more ambiguous grief and daily losses. It made it more difficult to do my grief work, to even have the capacity to revisit those hard places, but I knew it wouldn't disappear by ignoring it. I struggled with being the counselor who taught about grief yet still needed her own grief counseling.

It's incredibly hard to distill this long, roller-coaster ride of a journey into a few paragraphs. As I read back over these words, some of the sentences sound matter of fact, when in reality they were gut-wrenching. I felt the loss of hopes and dreams and experiences. I wished things could be different, like my mother-in-law meeting her grandchildren if we could have had them sooner. Some days I'd feel hopeful and strong, and some days I'd feel sideswiped. Sometimes, I was leveled with despair while wearing the responsibility of teaching my students how to help clients through it.

Now, after lots of personal work and with older children, I can see the benefits of this journey. I didn't want it, but I am a different kind of parent because of it. I have a lot of learned wisdom. I treasure my children in a different way because I had to wait so long. I share my journey in my classes freely now, because I want my students to recognize the strength that comes from our struggles. I tell my story because I want others to embrace the hard parts of their own stories and recognize that it can be a source of strength. I am so grateful for the lessons of the infertility journey while accepting the pain it brought.

SCHOLARSHIP AND SERVICE

As professors, we are evaluated based on our teaching, scholarship, and service. We've talked about ways to incorporate the concepts of the Hero's Journey into your classes, but maybe your knowledge of the Hero's Journey of infertility will become part of your research agenda. At the time of this writing, we could find no evidence of research, presentations, or professional development on the topic of counselor educator infertility, so you might be the one to help fill that gap.

If you are one of us, a counselor educator who experienced infertility, perhaps part of your Return phase will be through your service, using your painful journey to help others. You may start a support group, provide community education, or create a podcast. You might offer a class through your place of worship or provide the voice of an expert on a news program.

Obviously, we have a strong desire to help those hurting from reproductive loss issues. But, because the Hero's Journey is a universal one, this framework can be applied to other presenting concerns as well. The phases and stages are generally the same regardless of the reason for the journey, so, counselor educators, feel free to adapt it to your student's needs and your teaching strengths. You have many opportunities to apply what you have learned from the Hero's Journey to aid others through teaching, scholarship, and service.

Finally, we want to encourage you to honestly share your journey with your students when you are ready and when it is appropriate. Students taking their first steps into this profession have a strong desire to help others but a false belief that they need to have all their own problems solved first. They may even choose a helping profession to find answers during their own road of trials. Hearing a professor share the story of their own journey, and especially the resolution of the journey, regardless of the outcome, can be powerful in shaping the next generation of helpers. Use your complex emotional experiences when teaching about feelings identification in a skills course. Share your challenges to showing a childbirth video in a lifespan class. Discuss how infertility influenced your experience through grief stages.

Your role is such an important one, and we are grateful that you are willing to invest so much into your students' lives. If sharing your story is too painful, you aren't ready to tell it yet, or it isn't appropriate to do so, you can still express compassion. One of our professors showed a way to empathize without words. It was a touching gesture that maintained professionalism and required no self-disclosure. We'll leave you with this counselor educator's demonstration of empathy. One of us miscarried while working on her dissertation after ten years of not being able to conceive. We share that story now.

I was heartbroken, but I was determined to remain professional. In a meeting with my dissertation chair, Dr. Marianne Woodside, she asked how I was doing, and I burst into tears. I felt so ashamed, unprofessional, and incapable. As I sat, covered in embarrassment, she picked up a box of tissues, took one for herself, and handed the rest to me without saying a word. In that compassionate act, I knew she understood and cared. I don't know her story, but her response changed the way I now interact with my students. That day, I learned that empathy transcends words.

CONCLUSION

We wanted to write this book because we are counselor educators who have been on our own Hero's Journeys. We know the griefs, joys, hopes, disappointments, and social isolation firsthand. We know the challenges of bearing heavy, silent grief while teaching students to help their clients with their losses. And we know the critical importance of getting our own therapy and doing our own grief work. Even professionals need professional help at times. Our journeys have taken years, and they aren't complete yet. Because we are counselor educators, clinicians, supervisors, and now mothers, we want to pass on some practical help for professional helpers working with clients on this journey … and for those helpers that are walking this journey, too. That's our motivation. We hope we have been successful.

Now that you've read about the biopsychosocial crisis in Part One, explored who suffers from infertility in Part Two, and learned practical strategies and suggestions for helping in Part Three, we are at the end. Thank you for reading until the last page. We are three heroes who embarked on our own journeys. In the process, we were changed forever. Those you work with will be, too, but because they have you, their journeys can be resolved and become sources of strength.

REFERENCES

Centers for Disease Control and Prevention (2022). *Infertility FAQs*. Retrieved October 3, 2022 from https://www.cdc.gov/reproductivehealth/infertility/index.htm

Council for Accreditation of Counseling and Related Educational Programs (2015). *2016 CACREP standards*. Retrieved October 14, 2022, from http://www.cacrep.org/wp-content/uploads/2017/08/2016-Standards-with-citations.pdf

Jenkins, P. (2022, April 14). *How to Become a Sage*. Brilliantio. Retrieved October 3, 2022, from https://brilliantio.com/how-to-become-a-sage/

Hero's Journey Group Plan

Because of the isolating challenges of infertility, we believe that group therapy may be helpful for your clients, especially when combined with individual or couples therapy. To help you, we created a 12-session topic outline for leading a group on reproductive loss. We strongly recommend that you run it as a closed group so group members can get to know and trust each other over about three months.

Each session is structured to be part psychoeducational, imparting information about the Hero's Journey through infertility, and part support group, with discussion prompts. We encourage you to simply use this as a template and adapt it to best fit your leadership style and your group's needs. This group would work best with about 8–10 people with each weekly session lasting 1½ to 2 hours. You might run the group with women only or as a couple's group, so carefully consider how the dynamics and goals of the group might be different. We believe both would be helpful and needed. If you work with more specialized populations, such as those who are same-sex, adopting, or couples using surrogates, then consider specific groups for them, too, since one benefit of group support is to reduce isolation. Make sure you have written informed consent. Feel free to use this book as an optional supplemental reading so each group member can source additional information.

For each group session, we have provided an overview of the session, a warm-up activity, psychoeducation points, and discussion prompts. We strongly encourage you to combine the education portion with the discussion, allowing the group members to teach each other, but we have separated them here to clarify what you want to cover. Follow your own group leadership style, and use your strengths.

SUGGESTED GROUP PARAMETERS

Size: 8–10 people or 5 couples
Number of Sessions: 12
Length of Sessions: 1½ to 2 hours each

SESSION #1 – INTRODUCTIONS AND GROUP EXPECTATIONS

Obtain informed consent first.

Every group needs to begin with establishing some group norms. An essential norm in this group is the expectation that each member talks and shares honestly about their journey. The goals for this session are to create an open, safe environment and to facilitate group members starting to know and trust each other.

Warm Up

Begin the group with an activity of creating name tags or place cards so each member can visually see other members' names. Create something more permanent than a sticker so that you can collect them and use them again in the remaining sessions. It is harder to trust people who do not know your name.

Psychoeducation

Provide a visual of the Hero's Journey and briefly give an overview. See the handout at the end of this appendix (Figure A.1). The remainder of the group sessions will go into more depth. As participants answer these questions, it may help in the first session if you also answer them to create a culture of openness and sharing. Our preference is to introduce yourself first to help the group warm up and then answer the remaining questions last.

Discussion Prompts:

- Introduce yourself and tell us your favorite movie.
- If you are in a relationship, briefly tell us how you met and how long you have been together.
- Since this is a group about infertility, why did you decide to attend?
- What do you hope to get from this group?
- How did you feel coming into the group today? How has that changed now?

SESSION #2 – YOU ARE A HERO: THE HERO'S JOURNEY

Warm Up

Bring a cape. You can improvise by tying a blanket or sheet over the shoulders like you may have done as a child. Ask for a volunteer to wear the cape. After attaching the cape, proclaim that person a superhero and notice what happens next. Follow this with a discussion about what it means to be called a hero. If time allows you might want to ask if anyone else wants to be a hero and wear the cape to let other participants experience those feelings.

Psychoeducation

Explain the hero of the Hero's Journey, what the hero desires, and what the hero fears. This can be done through the discussion, with a little psychoeducation sprinkled in as needed.

Discussion Prompts:

- What did you notice when [the person's name] put on the hero's cape?
- How did their body language change?
- What did they say?
- How would you respond if I told you that you were the hero of your infertility story?
- What does it mean to be a hero?
- A hero in a story desires something. What do you desire on this journey?
- Heroes also fear things. What do you fear about the journey of infertility?
- The tension in the story comes from trying to balance desire and fear. How are you doing that? Which one seems to be winning?
- As you begin to see yourself as the hero of this story, what might be different this week?

SESSION #3 – THE SEPARATION PHASE

The first phase of the Hero's Journey is what brings the members of the group to the point of needing to set out on this journey. It includes everything that happened before that taught them lessons about the world, who or what controls what happens to them, and how to respond to obstacles. It is the growing discontent and what things they did in hopes that the problem would take care of itself. This phase of the journey shows how the hero separates from what was to the present reality of infertility.

Warm Up

Hand out blank paper and pens. If you don't have tables or desks available, you might need to provide a temporary writing surface as well. Ask group members to fold the paper in half and then in half again. When they unfold the paper, they should have four boxes. Label each box with one of the following headings and then give them 10 minutes to quickly write in whatever comes to mind. Tell them that they get to keep this paper and only share what is comfortable. They can add to it throughout the night and journal about it at home if they wish. We will reference this next week, too. In the four boxes, write:

- My Strengths
- Characteristics about Me that Limit Me
- What I Did to Attempt to Get Pregnant Before Seeing a Specialist
- How I Feel about Letting Go of What Life Was Like Before Infertility

Psychoeducation

Provide a brief explanation of the stages in the Separation Phase. Use the handout if it is helpful. Explain that this might not fit their story perfectly but that they will probably see some similarities with their story. These are the five stages:

- The Need for the Journey
- Resistance to the Journey
- Help and Hope
- The Point of No Return
- The Belly of the Whale

Discussion Prompts:

- Last week, we talked about the tension between what you desire and what you fear. How did that bring you to the point of needing this journey?
- How have you resisted this journey?
- What specifically motivates you to continue?
- Who are the people that provide help and hope for you?
- Did any of you have a point where you decided you were "all in" this journey? Maybe a time when you thought, "If I'm going to do this, then …"
- Who had a moment where you ran in the opposite direction to avoid this infertility journey? Or this might have been a time when you could have run in the opposite direction but decided not to run. Tell us about it.

SESSION #4 – THE QUEST PHASE

While all of this is a journey, the quest is to add a child to the family. The Separation Phase is everything that happens before it becomes a quest, and the Return Phase makes meaning out of the quest, but this phase is the emotional roller coaster of hope and despair. It is likely that this is where most of the group is on their own journeys, so the next five sessions will cover the stages that are part of this phase.

Warm Up

Ask the group to stand up and select a spot on an imaginary continuum line based on how they answer this question: Do you love or hate roller coasters? If they absolutely hate them and never ride any, they would stand on one side of the room, and if they are thrill-seekers who travel to ride even more intense coasters, they would stand on the opposite side. Everyone else picks a place somewhere in between. Ask why they chose to stand in the spot they picked. Afterward, they may return to their seats for the discussion.

Psychoeducation

Explain the stages of the Quest Phase. Learn about the struggles of members of the group, people that help on the journey, any temptations to give up, and beginning awareness that the journey might be bigger than the quest, and any insights or understandings they have learned. The stages of the Quest Phase are:

- Road of Trials
- Meeting the Guide
- The Temptation
- Atonement
- Climax of the Story
- The Ultimate Boon

Discussion Prompts:

- In the next few meetings, we'll go deeper into the stages of the Quest Phase, but today I want to give you an overview so we can keep the perspective of the journey. Let's begin with a quick round. Just give me a number from 1 to 10 (1 is easy, 10 is unbearably difficult) to indicate how hard this infertility journey has been for you.
- We started out today talking about roller coasters. That is a metaphor for the ups and downs of this journey. What kinds of things feel like the highs? What are the thrilling parts of this journey?

- Summarize the highs the group listed. It's important to realize that the highs are what keep us on the journey. That hope, the dream, the maybe-this-time optimism. We can soar with it. But then it drops, and you get jerked all over the place. Let's talk about the lows of the journey. What are some of yours?
- Have your lows ever gotten so intense that you wanted to quit the journey, even without a child?
- Some of you may like the variety of highs and lows (maybe less intense ones), but some of you may prefer a more even journey. How much control do you have over that?
- What can you do to have more control over your journey?
- What is your biggest takeaway from this meeting?

SESSION #5 – GRIEVING THE LOSSES

This session explores grief, loss, and the concept of disenfranchised grief. Make sure that you have tissue available as this session could be heavy and painful. Some members may vocalize losses for the first time, making them feel more real. Some will label grief in new ways. Some will express anger, which may mask the deeper grief. Convey plenty of empathy, and use reflecting statements to help your group express their grief.

Warm Up

The following paragraphs are a sample script. Pause after each sentence to give group members time to do what you ask. Use a quieter, but still easily heard, voice. You might want to add music. The point of the exercise is to use the senses to ground the group members in the present moment and space. If anyone becomes dysregulated later during the discussion, you can come back to this to help them regulate.

We are going to talk about grief and loss today, so this meeting might be really hard for some of you. Before we begin, I'd like to do a quick grounding exercise to help us prepare. We're going to face some enemies in your journey today, and you might not feel ready for the battle. That's okay and normal. If we need to pull back, I'll help you do that. I am one of your guides on this journey.

Right now, I'd like you to put both feet on the floor and notice the solid place beneath your feet. Push your feet down to really feel it … Good. Now, look around this room for the color blue. Just notice anything you see that is blue. What I am going to do is walk you through using a few of your senses to become present right here in this room … You may have come from work, experienced traffic getting here, or have other life stressors, but for the next few minutes, I want to invite you to let go of all of it and just be here.

If you are comfortable closing your eyes, go ahead and do that … Take a few deep breaths … As you exhale, think the word, "Relax … " Now, notice any sensations in your body. Notice the temperature of your hands … any tightness in your forehead … and any sensations in your abdomen. Now, let's turn to the sense of hearing. What do you hear right now? … As we finish this short exercise, I want you to again push down with your feet and feel the ground. Notice the chair you are sitting on … Take a final deep breath and open your eyes when you are ready.

As we talk tonight, if it starts to feel too overwhelming, just take a deep breath and look around for the color blue. Then, push your feet down to feel the floor. I'll be watching, but please let me know if you feel overwhelmed. You are not alone on this journey.

Psychoeducation

The Hero's Journey of infertility has many losses. Some may experience deaths of hoped-for children through stillbirth or miscarriage, but those deaths may not be recognized by others as losses. Some may have lost children through failed adoptions, foster children who moved to different homes, or other family members' children they hoped to raise. Most of this group is grieving hoped-for children that never happened. They lost dreams, anticipated ceremonies, and expectations. Many have lost a sense of control over their lives, and friends who moved on to the baby stage of life and feeling normal. Disenfranchised grief is an unrecognized grief, and your group has many of those. The goal of this session is to begin to identify these things as losses and grief as a natural part of the healing process.

Discussion Prompts:

- Loss. As I look around the room, I know that we have a lot of losses around infertility. When the loss is yours, it's very painful, so avoid comparing your loss to others in the group. What are some of the losses you have experienced, big and small?
- What was the response of people around you when you experienced these losses?
- When you have a loss, whether it is a person, an abstract thing, or something invisible, a natural part of that experience is grief. We grieve in lots of different ways. How do you grieve?
- What are some of the invisible things you grieve? (Examples: the dream of a growing family, having a deceased parent at the birth of your baby, baby

showers with your current group of friends, kids growing up together, invasive medical procedures, etc.)

- Sometimes, you find people who get it when you have a loss, but sometimes, people around you don't get it at all. This is called disenfranchised grief. What was it like for you when people around you didn't get it?
- How does labeling your sadness, anger, disappointment, coping behaviors, and other things as grief change things?
- What can you do to allow yourself to grieve, yet also care for yourself this week?

SESSION #6 – THE ROAD OF TRIALS STAGE

This session builds community through shared challenges and provides a safe place for group members to talk about the difficult part of the journey. Kulikov (2021) has created a thorough mind map, which would make an excellent handout for this discussion after the warm-up exercise. You can access it at: https://digitalcommons.unf.edu/soars/2021/spring_2021/28/

Warm Up

Last week we talked about the losses of infertility and the need to grieve those losses. Loss is one of the challenges – or battles, to use our Hero's Journey language – of infertility, but we face battles on many fronts. Today, we are going to make a mind map of your battles. I'd like you to take a piece of paper and draw a rectangle in the middle. Inside the rectangle, write the word *infertility*. Now, you are going to draw six circles around the rectangle that you connect with a line to start your mind map. Label them: *physical, emotional, mental, social, spiritual*, and *financial*. You probably have battles in all these areas. Maybe you can think of other categories, too. Start with these, but feel free to add others that apply to you. I want you to map as many battles in each of these areas as you can that apply to your own personal journey. You are going to keep this paper, and you do not need to share anything on it that you don't want to share. We'll take about 10 minutes to do this …

You will probably think of others as we continue our discussion, so feel free to keep adding things as you think of them. To keep us on track, though, we're going to move on to the discussion.

Psychoeducation

Explore the many kinds of trials that come with this journey, especially in the categories of physical, emotional, mental, social, spiritual, and financial. Many of the trials will come up in the discussion, but feel free to add others. Here are some examples: anxiety, loss of identity, shame and stigma, lack of family support, fear, relationship strain, losses (hope, meaning in life, dreams, parents, babies), stress, embarrassing medical treatments, pain, injustice, financial strain, spiritual crisis, etc.

Discussion Prompts:

- What would you say has been the biggest battle on your journey so far?
- What did you write on your mind map that surprised you or was unexpected?
- Which category has the most battles for you?
- What are your weapons for fighting these battles? Where do you get them?
- Unfortunately, you don't always get to fight one battle at a time. Sometimes, you have these things coming at you from all sides. Which ones seem to occur at the same time?
- Now, you have this list of many of the things you face on the road of trials. What do you want to do with it?

SESSION #7 – GUIDES AND TEMPTERS

Part of the Hero's Journey is the characters who step in and out of the story. These aren't the sidekicks who travel alongside the hero but those who are briefly part of the story yet may have a big impact. You, the helping professional, are a guide in the story, and other members of the group may also be guides. There are also tempters who make the journey more painful or try to get the hero to quit the quest. Be cautious about labeling people as tempters, but be candid that they offer temptation. For example, it won't be helpful to label the mother-in-law as a temptress when she brings up the waste of money on fertility treatments that might not work, but it is very appropriate to say that it brings up the temptation to just give up and not risk more family gossip and financial stress.

Warm Up

Give every group member two pieces of candy: a candy kiss and a piece of sour candy. Explain that some people that we meet on the journey are helpful. They provide a pick-me-up, encouraging words, or a shoulder to cry on. They may point you in a new direction or help in other ways. They are like these candy kisses, and we are going to call them guides. Go ahead and eat the kiss, if you want.

Others sour our journey with hurtful words, discouragement, and shame. Sometimes they don't mean it that way or even realize it. Others might enjoy pulling you down. These people make the journey harder, and you may consider quitting the journey after interacting with these people because it seems like it would be less painful. We're not going to call these people tempters because that might cause you trouble at your next family gathering, but we are going to recognize the temptation. We are going to label *things* as tempters. Some things offer short-term relief, but later, we feel guilt, remorse, or self-loathing because it risks what we really want. Food, alcohol, substance use, gaming, avoidance, procrastination, and others could be tempters.

Psychoeducation

Define the words *guides* and *temptations*. A guide is someone who shows the way or provides assistance. A temptation offers short-term relief but threatens the quest. This session helps the group identify their own guides and temptations.

Discussion Prompts:

- We are now more than halfway through our group, so let's talk about people that have been helpful. Who has helped you, in big or small ways? How were they helpful?
- Where did you expect help but were disappointed?
- You might not want to say these out loud, but who are the sour candies that you've encountered on the journey?
- A temptation offers short-term relief but threatens your quest to have a baby. What are your temptations?
- This journey brings a tremendous amount of pain. Remember the mind maps we made? You will naturally try things to reduce the pain, and you will keep doing those things if they work, even if it is short-term and threatens what you really want. Sometimes, you just want to not hurt for a while. How can you care for yourself while resisting these tempters?
- How does it help to identify guides, tempters, and temptations?

SESSION #8 – PLOT TWIST

At some point in the journey, the hero recognizes that the journey is bigger than she is. This is the transformational atonement stage. Your group members may not have reached this point yet, so it might be helpful to address this as something to anticipate. Also, some of these difficult questions may not yet have answers. Assure them that it is okay not to know, but wrestling with the questions is part of the journey.

Warm Up

Lead a discussion with this prompt: What are some of the best movie or book plot twists of all time?

Psychoeducation

The goal of this session is to begin to make sense of the pain of infertility. The atonement stage of the quest phase is a pivotal plot point when the hero understands the true purpose of her journey was not simply the quest to have a baby. It's much bigger. It may include that child's life and all the lives that intersect with it. This is the peak of the hero's transformation as she faces the conflict with the person or entity that holds power in her life. This stage is often spiritual and existential, but unlike previous wrestling with these questions, they find answers here, including a higher purpose in suffering.

Discussion Prompts:

- What would you say if I told you that the Hero's Journey isn't about having a baby? It's much bigger than that. How would you respond?
- We're going to get a little deep today. Some of you aren't quite at this stage of the Hero's Journey yet, and that's okay. You'll know what to anticipate in the future. In the atonement stage of the journey, you begin to find some answers. This journey has been painful, so what is the purpose of that pain?
- How do you explain how good things might come out of this?
- Who or what do you believe has control over this journey? Why is pain part of the process?
- How might the timing of having your baby be right on schedule? Who is impacted by when a baby is born?
- What are some other lessons you have learned so far on your journey?
- What is it like to wrestle with these hard questions?
- Are there any parallels between your story and some of the plot twists we talked about earlier?
- This session was a lot deeper, so let's lighten things up before we go home. What is something that made you laugh or smile this week?

SESSION #9 – APOTHEOSIS/ CLIMAX OF THE STORY

This session is about the final battle, facing the possibility that the quest may not end like the group members want. Now that you have spent eight sessions talking about the hopes, the griefs, and the higher purpose in the journey, in this session they will face their fears around what happens if they don't get what they desire. Hopefully, your group has well-established norms of safety, but it will be important to remind them. Their fears may not be politically correct or socially acceptable, so it is essential to have a safe place to express them as their personal fears.

Warm Up

Fold a piece of paper in half and turn it to look like a book. Instruct group members to write the title "My Story" and decorate the front like a book, if they wish. Then, ask them to open the "book" and write three paragraphs. The first paragraph is the ending they want for their story. The second is an ending they don't want but could live with. The third paragraph would be the worst ending possible, the one they don't want to even think about. Start the discussion prompts after this activity.

Psychoeducation

Regardless of the actual family result, in this stage, the hero makes peace with (and wins ultimate victory over) infertility. This stage helps her find a personal and individual answer, so she can ultimately succeed in healing from the journey.

Discussion Prompts:

- Let's face the final ending of your quest to have children today. What is the happy ending you described in your first paragraph?
- I hope you all get the happy ending, but the reality is that even *Frozen* had a sequel that showed it wasn't all rainbows and butterflies and happily ever after. So, what did you write in your not-perfect-but-livable paragraph?
- Now, let's face the villains, your fears. What is the worst that could happen? What makes that so frightening?
- What was it like to say those fears out loud? How do you feel about it now?
- We've been fighting a difficult battle in this session. Fighting your worst fears is the climax of the story. I want you to physically lay down your imaginary weapons now. Put them on the floor. You did it. It's probably not your last fight, but by addressing it directly, you faced it. How are you doing now?

SESSION #10 – RETURN AND HEALING

Too many travelers on the infertility journey quit when the quest ends (with a child or not) and miss the critical healing part of the journey. They spend years distracting themselves and avoiding what is unresolved. In this session, your group will learn about acceptance. Again, most of your group may still be in the quest phase, so you want to encourage them to see the journey through to the end.

Warm Up

You all know each other well by now. Today, I want to give you a chance to say something to someone else in the group that you haven't said yet.

Psychoeducation

Your group must reassemble into a life changed. In the Return Phase, the consuming focus is no longer on having a baby, and the hero is not the same person she was when she started this journey. The journey has brought many emotions, but some of those are probably not yet resolved. This is also a time to make peace with the consequences of career and life decisions made during the journey.

Discussion Prompts:

- I'm glad you came back after the last couple of sessions. We got into the messy parts of the journey. Now, let's start putting it back together. What are a few things in your journey that still aren't resolved?
- If you could start this journey over, what would you do differently?
- Have you made any career or life decisions during this journey that had consequences, positive or negative? What were they?
- What do you still need?
- How have you changed? How can those changes become strengths?
- We only have two more sessions left. What do you have now that you didn't have before starting this group?

SESSION #11 – FREEDOM TO LIVE

This is next to the last session, and the last stage of the Hero's Journey of infertility. It is a place of acceptance, even if the quest didn't end the way the hero hoped. It is a time of moving on, leaving the pain, money, medical procedures, rollercoaster emotions, and efforts needed. In this stage, the hero can recognize her growth and even some benefits of the journey, but she can also acknowledge the difficulty of the road of trials. She may decide to use what she has learned to help others and become a guide.

Warm Up

Draw a picture of what freedom after the infertility journey looks like for you. You can draw symbols, stick people, abstract shapes, or whatever works. It doesn't matter how artistic it is. I just want you to think about the idea of freedom and what that means for you.

Psychoeducation

This stage is the last one on the hero's journey of infertility. After a difficult journey, she has finally earned the freedom to live in comfort and peace. If processed to completion, she arrives at a place of acceptance. There may be other journeys (after all, good stories have sequels), but this one can end with a satisfying, if not perfect, ending.

Discussion Prompts:

- We've made it to the last stage of the hero's journey. For most of you, you aren't quite here yet, but I want you to have hope that it is coming. All your hard work is going to pay off. The last stage is called, "Freedom to Live." You drew some things to show what this is for you. Who would like to share what they drew?
- Other words we could use for freedom are acceptance or resolution. Let's break this down into specific areas of our lives. What would resolution feel like physically? Mentally? Socially? Emotionally? Spiritually? Financially?
- Which of those areas do you think will be the hardest for you to get to?
- A couple of sessions ago, we talked about our biggest fears. How can you get to a place of peace, acceptance, and resolution even if the worst outcome happens?
- How is it possible to grieve so many losses on this journey and yet still be able to feel joy?
- We all want to just get to this stage. Wouldn't that be great? Why do you think the journey requires so many stages before you can experience the freedom to live?
- Next week is our last session. I thought it would be fun to celebrate all the work we've done together and how far you've come in this group.

How would you like to do that? (Ideas: bring a dish for a meal together, have a dessert bar, write notes to each other, givebacks to the group which is described in the warm-up of session #12, etc.)

SESSION #12 – ENDING

This session is a celebration of the journey of the group. During these 12 meetings, the group members have likely had victories and defeats and journeyed through them together. This meeting, like all endings, reviews your past together, how far you have come, and then prepares for the future.

Warm Up

Givebacks are a way of saying thank you to the group for their contributions during this group experience. This can be a highly meaningful closure activity. Allow each member a brief time to express their gratitude to individuals or the whole group.

Note: if you suggest this in the previous meeting, some might enjoy preparing small gifts, snacks, or writing thoughtful notes. It works well if you leave it open for them to express gratitude in whatever unique ways they want or by simply saying, "Thanks" with no preparation at all.

Second Note: Emphasize that the sharing time needs to be brief. Consider how much time you have for this activity and how many people will share and suggest no longer than that many minutes.

Psychoeducation

Review the Hero's Journey and your group's journey.

Discussion Prompts:

- We did it! We have come to the end of this group. Do you remember your first few minutes sitting together in this room of strangers? What was that like?
- How are you different now?
- We've spent a while talking about the Hero's Journey. Let's review the phases of the journey. What do you remember about the Separation Phase? The Quest Phase? The Return Phase?
- This group has been meaningful to me, too. I have enjoyed watching your progress and felt so proud of you as you worked through the difficult parts. (Add appropriate self-disclosure here.)

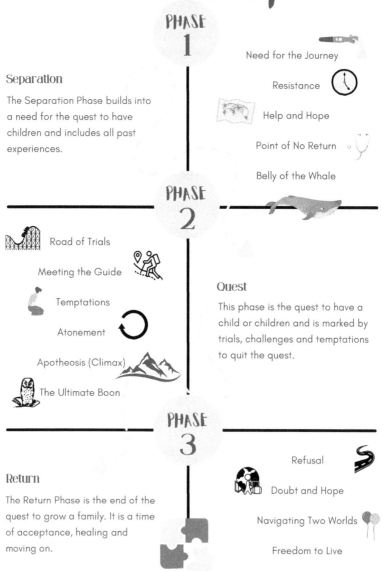

The Hero's Journey of Infertility

PHASE 1

Separation

The Separation Phase builds into a need for the quest to have children and includes all past experiences.

Need for the Journey

Resistance

Help and Hope

Point of No Return

Belly of the Whale

PHASE 2

Road of Trials

Meeting the Guide

Temptations

Atonement

Apotheosis (Climax)

The Ultimate Boon

Quest

This phase is the quest to have a child or children and is marked by trials, challenges and temptations to quit the quest.

PHASE 3

Refusal

Doubt and Hope

Navigating Two Worlds

Freedom to Live

Return

The Return Phase is the end of the quest to grow a family. It is a time of acceptance, healing and moving on.

FIGURE A.1 Handout for the Hero's Journey of Infertility

- Before we finish, I want to talk about what happens next. Some of you may realize that you need more personal or couples' counseling. [Provide referral options, support group information, and contact information here.]
- So, let's bring our time together to a close with this last discussion question. What is a highlight from our time together in this group?

REFERENCE

Kulikov, E. (2021). Psychosocial effect of infertility and what counselors and others can do about it. [Poster presentation]. Retrieved October 21, 2022, from https://digitalcommons.unf.edu/soars/2021/spring_2021/28/

Seven Types of Conflict

In literary terms, there are seven types of plot conflicts. Your client will likely experience several kinds of these, so becoming familiar with them will aid in your work. Some clients might appreciate carrying the story metaphor further and overtly labeling their experiences this way, but others might not, so follow your client's preferences. Either way, it will help you to understand whether the conflict arises internally or externally. These are the types of conflict:

1. **Hero vs. Character(s)** – Your client may disagree with her partner about what to do next, how far medical interventions should go, or going deeper into debt. She may also experience jealousy of a best friend's happy pregnancy or frustration with a mother's unsolicited suggestions. She may be angry at her doctor's misrepresentation of what would happen or at a teen couple in the waiting room giggling over an ultrasound. Character vs. character conflicts may be short-term or stretch on for years.

2. **Hero vs. Society** – Despite shifts in public opinion that allow more variability than in past centuries, women feel pressure to marry and have children in conventional ways following a conventional timeline. Those experiencing infertility are usually out of step with those expectations, and the longer they struggle with it, the more unacceptable they may feel. This may even result in shaming, blaming, and accusing her. It most certainly adds to her isolation and feeling misunderstood. If the hero is part of any minority subculture, she will also likely experience this conflict.

3. **Hero vs. Nature** – She may wonder why her body will not work correctly and learn more about her reproductive system than she ever expected. The natural methods of procreation have proved unsuccessful, and the hero

may wonder about environmental toxins, chemicals in her food, bleach in feminine products, her own in-utero exposures, and countless other things that she believes may have caused or contributed to this problem. For many of these things, she may have suspicions, but no evidence to confirm or dismiss them, so she is left to speculate in ambiguity.

4. **Hero vs. Technology** – The science around medical interventions for infertility is astounding. Embryos can be created in labs with a sperm and an egg. They may be retrieved from the client and her partner, but either or both may be donated from another who is known or anonymous. The pregnant woman may be your client or a surrogate. Medication stimulates ovulation, sperm motility, and even lactation for an adoptive mom. The chance for multiples increases, even for rare quadruplets and quintuplets. The science is marvelous but also murky with legal, ethical, and religious implications. The decisions made with today's information may impact generations. For example, the surge in DNA testing means identifying donors who may have thought they were anonymous or finding previously unknown siblings.

5. **Hero vs. Supernatural** – It is impossible to deal with life and death without considering existential questions. Are medical interventions going too far in "playing God?" Is conception merely chance or orchestrated by a higher being? If the client believes in God (or another deity), does He care about her suffering? Is He withholding life from her? Is she being punished or growing through a challenge? Whose fault is this suffering? Who can relieve it? Do not be afraid to explore your client's faith and beliefs.

6. **Hero vs. Fate** – This may be related to her views on the Supernatural, but part of her journey may seem inevitable and unavoidable. This conflict is about free will and autonomy, both of which are threatened by infertility. The hero may not feel like she has many choices, and she may not feel much control over the situation.

7. **Hero vs. Self** – The final type of conflict is her battle with herself. She may despise herself for her past decisions, her poor nutrition choices, and living in a body that is letting her down. She may fight herself physically, mentally, and emotionally, and even engage in behaviors to punish herself. It may seem like her own nature is polarized and her own body is the enemy.

As you hear your client's story, you will likely identify several of these conflicts. Listen for patterns that indicate recurring conflicts in one or more of these categories, which may suggest a need to focus therapeutic work on that type of conflict. In general, clients will experience a growing discomfort in the Separation Phase, possible distress in the Quest Phase, and acceptance and resolution of the conflict in the Return Phase.

Glossary

Abbreviated Grief a type of grief that passes relatively quickly or more quickly than expected

Abortion a medical procedure that uses medication or surgery to remove an embryo or fetus and placenta from the uterus

Absent Grief an experience in which someone doesn't experience any type of grief

Ambiguous Grief a type of grief in which there is a lack of information or closure surrounding the loss

Anxiety an emotion characterized by feelings of worry, nervousness, or unease

Anticipatory Grief a type of grief in which the loss was imminent, and the person grieved in anticipation

Azoospermia a condition diagnosed when no sperm are produced

Bereavement a state or condition of having experienced a loss which is often associated with a specific time period, usually when sadness and pain are at their highest levels

Biopsychosocial a term used to describe the association between biological, psychological, and social factors related to a variety of topics

Chemical Pregnancy a pregnancy that ends before the fifth week; a type of miscarriage, but often with no symptoms because the embryo forms and may even implant but then stops developing

Chronic Grief a type of grief characterized by prolonged or extremely intense grief

Chronic Sorrow   a reaction to losses that are not final and continue to be present in the life of the griever

Complicated Grief   a type of grief that occurs when a response to loss differs significantly from normal expectations

Concentration of Sperm   a term used to describe the number of sperm

Conception   a process that occurs when an egg is released from a woman's ovary, travels down the fallopian tubes, joins with sperm, and implants in the lining of the uterus

Delayed Grief   a type of grief that occurs much later than expected and tends to manifest itself when people suppress the pain associated with the loss

Depression   an emotion characterized by a depressed mood, loss of interest in daily activities, and a sense of hopelessness and helplessness

Dilation and Evacuation   a type of abortion procedure used for pregnancy termination between 13 and 21 weeks.

Diminished Ovarian Reserve   a condition in which not enough eggs are present due to aging

Disenfranchised Grief   a type of grief that occurs when the loss is not societally recognized or acknowledged

Early Infant Death   also called neonatal death, is a type of death that occurs within the first 28 days of life

Ectopic Pregnancy   a pregnancy in which implantation of the fertilized egg occurs outside the uterus

Egg Donation   donated eggs are combined with a partner's sperm and then the embryos are placed in the uterus

Embryo Donation   individuals adopt embryos that have been frozen by other people

Frozen Embryo Transfer   thawing and transfer of frozen embryos

Functional Hypothalamic Amenorrhea   the cessation of menstruation, which is caused by excessive exercise, weight loss, and/or stress associated with anorexia nervosa

Gamete Intrafallopian Transfer   a type of assisted reproductive technology in which sperm and eggs are mixed together and then inserted into the fallopian tubes in hopes fertilization will occur

Grief   an emotion characterized by deep sorrow, particularly related to a death or loss

Hysteroscopy   a minimally invasive surgical procedure that investigates potential abnormalities or irregularities with the reproductive organs, especially the uterine cavity

Hysterosalpingogram   a type of test that involves injecting fluid into the uterus and fallopian tubes to check for blockages, especially blockages in the fallopian tubes

Identity   the distinguished personality or character of an individual

In Vitro Fertilization   a type of assisted reproductive technology that involves combining sperm and eggs in a laboratory and then placing the embryos in the uterus three to five days after fertilization

Infertility   a condition diagnosed when pregnancy is not achieved within one year of unprotected intercourse or one year of therapeutic donor insemination; for those over 35 years of age, the time frame is six months

Infertility-Specific Distress   the degree of emotional strain that is associated with an inability to conceive or experience childbirth

Intersectional Discrimination   when two or more multiple grounds operate simultaneously and interact in an inseparable manner, producing distinct and specific forms of discrimination

Intrauterine Insemination   a type of treatment for infertility that can be used in conjunction with ovulation induction; involves placing sperm directly into the uterus with a small catheter

Laparoscopy   a minimally invasive surgical procedure that investigates potential abnormalities or irregularities with the reproductive organs, especially the outside of the uterus, ovaries, fallopian tubes, and internal pelvic area

Late-term Abortion   also called intact dilation and extraction, is a type of abortion procedure that terminates a pregnancy between 20 and 24 weeks

Medical Abortion   the use of medications to end a pregnancy of 10 weeks or less

Miscarriage   the spontaneous loss of a pregnancy before the 20th week; the most common type of pregnancy loss

Morphology   a term used to describe the shape of sperm

Motility   a term used to describe the movement of sperm

Mourning   the expression of deep sorrow shown by someone who is grieving; often characterized by an outward expression of sadness that is action-oriented

Ovulation Induction   a type of treatment for infertility in which medications are used to stimulate egg production in the ovaries

Ovulation Disorders   disorders caused by problems with the regulation of reproductive hormones which affect egg production and release

Premature Birth   a birth that occurs prior to the 37th week of pregnancy

Prolonged Grief Disorder   a disorder that is diagnosed when at least one year has passed since a loss has occurred and begins to interfere with daily functioning

Polycystic Ovarian Syndrome   a hormonal disorder causing enlarged ovaries with small cysts on the outer edges

Premature Ovarian Insufficiency   a condition in which the ovaries stop working normally before the age of 40

Prostaglandins Abortion   a type of abortion that terminates a pregnancy in the second trimester and uses hormones causing uterine contractions

Post-traumatic Stress Disorder   disorder diagnosed when a person has trouble recovering from experiencing or witnessing a traumatic event that included feelings of fear, helplessness, and/or horror

Primary Infertility   type of infertility diagnosed when a couple has never conceived

Recurrent Pregnancy Loss   a condition diagnosed when two or more miscarriages have occurred

Reproductive Endocrinologist   a gynecologist with specialized training in both male and female infertility issues as well as recurrent pregnancy loss

Scrotal Ultrasound   a test conducted to assess problems in the testicles

Secondary Infertility   type of infertility diagnosed when people achieved pregnancy at least once but then are unable to conceive again

Secondary Loss   a type of loss that occurs when a primary loss triggers subsequent losses

Semen Analysis   a test conducted to determine sperm count, shape, and/or movement.

Sonohysterogram   a type of test that involves injecting fluid into the uterus and fallopian tubes to check for blockages, especially blockages in the uterine cavity

Special Needs Diagnosis   the diagnosis of a variety of conditions including birth defects, disabilities, or terminal illness

Sperm Donation   donated sperm which are combined with a partner's eggs and then the embryos are placed in the uterus

Sterilization   a permanent form of birth control

Stillbirth   the loss of a baby at or after the 20th week either before or during delivery

Surrogacy   a type of assisted reproduction where couples work with a gestational surrogate who will carry and care for their baby until birth

Therapeutic Donor Insemination   a type of artificial insemination that uses donor sperm from someone who is either anonymous or known

Transvaginal Ultrasound   a procedure that examines organs such as the bladder, uterus, vagina, and fallopian tubes; sound waves bounce off organs inside the pelvis from an instrument that has been inserted into the vagina

Traumatic Grief   a type of grief that occurs when the manner of the loss was perceived to be horrifying, unexpected, violent, and/or traumatic

Tubal Ligation   a form of sterilization that closes off the fallopian tubes and prevents the egg from traveling down the fallopian tubes and the sperm from reaching the egg

Unexplained Infertility   a type of infertility diagnosed when no cause is determined

Vacuum Aspiration   a type of abortion procedure used to terminate a pregnancy between seven and twelve weeks

Varicocele   a condition that involves swelling of the veins in the testicles that may impact sperm quality and quantity

Vasectomy   a procedure that involves tying, cutting, clipping, or sealing the tube that carries sperm from the testicles

Zygote Intrafallopian Transfer   a type of assisted reproductive technology in which sperm and eggs are combined in a lab and then introduced into the fallopian tubes within 24 hours

Index

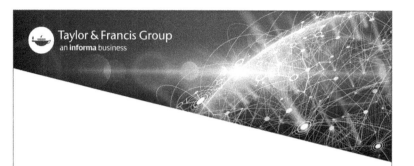

For Product Safety Concerns and Information please contact our EU
representative GPSR@taylorandfrancis.com
Taylor & Francis Verlag GmbH, Kaufingerstraße 24, 80331 München, Germany

www.ingramcontent.com/pod-product-compliance
Ingram Content Group UK Ltd.
Pitfield, Milton Keynes, MK11 3LW, UK
UKHW021449080625
459435UK00012B/426